Canadian Pharmacy Exams

Pharmacy Technician OSPE Workbook

Dr. Fatima S. Marankan

Phi Publishing

Canadian Pharmacy Exams – Pharmacy Technician OSPE Workbook

Pharmacy is an ever-changing science. As new research and clinical experience broaden our knowledge, changes in treatment and drug therapy are needed. The author and contributors of Canadian Pharmacy Exams – Pharmacy Technician OSPE Workbook have checked with resources believed to be reliable in their efforts to provide information that is complete and generally in accord with the standards accepted at the time of publication. However, in view of the possibility of human error or changes in medical sciences, neither the author nor any other party who has been involved in the preparation or publication of this work warrants that the information contained herein is in every respect accurate or complete and they disclaim all responsibility for any errors or omissions or for the results obtained from the use of the information contained in this work.

Library and Archives Canada Cataloguing in Publication

Phi Publishing
Canadian Pharmacy Exams Pharmacy Technician OSPE Workbook / Author, Dr. Fatima S. Marankan – 1st Canadian Edition.

About the Author

Dr. Marankan holds a postgraduate degree in pharmacy from the College of Pharmacy at UIC, USA coupled with extensive experience in pharmacy instruction at the University of British Columbia, Canada. Dr. Marankan was recently a visiting medical professor. Her academic, research and teaching achievements have been recognized by the Paul Sang Award at the University of Illinois at Chicago and the TLEF Award at the University of British Columbia, Canada. Furthermore, Dr. Marankan was the lead consultant in the development and implementation of OSCE training in Vancouver, Canada.

Throughout her education and career as pharmacy instructor at the University of British Columbia, Fatima has gained extensive understanding of the requirements of pharmacy licensing exams in Canada. This knowledge has guided the development of the Canadian Pharmacy Exams Series:

- Pharmacist Evaluating Exam Practice - Volume 1
- Pharmacist Evaluating Exam Practice – Volume 2
- Pharmacist MCQ Review
- Pharmacist OSCE Workbook
- Pharmacy Technician MCQ Review
- Pharmacy Technician OSPE Workbook

Thank you to all contributing reviewers!

Preface

The regulation of pharmacy technicians in Canada has led to an expanded scope of practice. Despite some variations from jurisdiction to jurisdiction, the core nine competencies of pharmacy technicians practice identified by the National Association of Pharmacy Regulatory Authorities (NAPRA) remain consistent nationally. In order to become regulated (certified) a pharmacy technician must satisfy the requirements of the Pharmacy Examining Board of Canada (PEBC) by completing successfully the Qualifying Exam divided in Part 1: MCQ (questions) and Part 2: OSPE (stations) to ensure pharmacy technicians have the necessary entry-level professional knowledge, skills and abilities to work effectively and safely within their scope of practice. The following core nine competencies of pharmacy technician practice, represent the keystones of the Qualifying Exam:

1. Ethical, Legal and Professional Responsibilities
2. Patient Care
3. Product Distribution
4. Practice Setting
5. Health Promotion
6. Knowledge and Research Application

Pharmacy technicians and pharmacists work as a team to ensure optimal delivery of drug therapy. To that end, pharmacy technicians are primarily responsible for the technical aspects of a prescription whereas pharmacists focus on its clinical implications. Both groups assume responsibility for their own actions, contribute to the overall functioning of the pharmacy, and are accountable to the public.

A candidate for OSPE Exam must be prepared to demonstrate practical skills in interactive and non-interactive stations. Stations are designed to evaluate several skills such as:

- Gathering information from a Standardized Patient, Standardized Client or Standardized Health Professional to solve a drug-related problem
- Gathering information from a Standardized Patient, Standardized Client or Standardized Health Professional to solve an ethical issue
- Addressing the questions of a Standardized Patient, Standardized Client or Standardized Health Professional
- Making a referral when appropriate
- Screen and evaluate new prescriptions
- Document information in a patient record
- Check the accuracy of patient records
- Check the accuracy of prepared medications
- Update a patient record
- Check the accuracy of prepared/compounded medications
- Check the accuracy of compounding techniques
- Compound a product

Canadian Pharmacy Exams™ - Pharmacy Technician OSPE Workbook is designed as a self-study or group-study tool to help the student seeking pharmacy technician certification in Canada test his/her exam readiness, identify areas of strength and weakness. The book provides an extensive opportunity to test and improve relevant practical skills within the nine competencies listed above. The book contains a mix of interactive stations, non-interactive stations (prescription and dispensed product check, MAR-blister pack check, compounding skills), medication reconciliation chart, answer forms and candidate assessment sheets.

All stations are supplemented by detailed solutions and explanations to ensure further understanding and learning of new concepts. These comments are truly the keystone of Canadian Pharmacy Exams™. We trust that each Canadian Pharmacy Exams™ book is a valuable learning and self-assessment tool towards Canadian Pharmacy Licensure or Canadian Pharmacy Technician Certification/Regulation. The following book is also available at Amazon: **Canadian Pharmacy Exams™ Pharmacy Technician MCQ Review**

Trusted Convenient Comprehensive Canadian Pharmacy Exams™ Online Review for Pharmacists and Technicians at www.cpepreponline.com

CCCEP Accredited Pharmacy Technician Regulation Review. Earn 6 CCCEP CEUs
FREE Computer-Based Exam Readiness Tests
FREE Pharmacy Resources

References

Compendium of Therapeutic Choices, 2019
Compendium of Pharmaceuticals and Specialties, 2019
Compendium of Products for Minor Ailments, 2019
Rx Files, 2017
Workbook for the Manual for Pharmacy Technicians, 2013
Pharmacology for Pharmacy Technicians, 2012
Complete Math Review for the Pharmacy Technician, 2014
Compounding Guidelines for Pharmacies, 2014
Martindale The Complete Drug Reference, 2017
Pharmacoethics A Problem-Based Approach, 2003
Communication Skills in Pharmacy Practice, 2011

Content

HOW TO USE OSPE WORKBOOK

Interactive Stations

Self-Study Option

You have 6 minutes to complete each station. Time yourself!

1. Make sure to have access to suggested reference(s) for the station.
2. As a replacement for Candidate Notebook, a Station Review Form is added to each station. Use the form to write useful notes as you review the station. For self-study, you may use the same form to show how you would solve the case.
3. Review the Solution following the completion of the station. Compare the Solution to your Station Review Form to evaluate your performance.

Practice, Practice, Practice …

Group-Study Option

A group of three candidates is suggested.

You have 6 minutes to complete each station.

1. Assign each candidate to one of the following three roles:

- OSPE Candidate. Have a copy of Candidate Instructions including Patient Profile, if available, Station Review Form (Candidate Notebook). Have access to suggested reference(s) for the station.
- Standardized Patient (SP), Standardized Client (SC) or Standardized Health Professional (SHP) depending on the station. Have a copy of SP, SC or SHP Instructions including Patient Profile if available.
- OSPE Assessor. Have a copy of the Assessment Form and Solution to evaluate the candidate. Time the candidate!

2. Review and discuss the Solution following the completion of the station.

Practice, Practice, Practice …

Important Tip: Make sure to use role reversal by playing the patient at least twice. Role reversal is a powerful technique proven to enhance the counselling skills of healthcare professionals. It improves significantly your understanding of patient expectations and concerns.

Non-interactive Stations

Non-Interactive Stations include:

Prescription and Dispensed Product Check
MAR (Medication Administration Record) - Blister Pack Check
Compounding Skills

You have 6 minutes to complete each station. Time yourself!

Make sure you have a recent copy of Compendium of Pharmaceuticals and Specialties (CPS)

Use the Answer Form to record your answers.

Review the Answer Key following the completion of the station.

Evaluate for performance.

Medication Reconciliation Chart

Patient information - Full name - Birthdate - Address **Medical History** - Health conditions - Allergies (symptoms, causes/triggers…)	**Ask about all medications (Rx and non-Rx)** - Prescription - Over-the-counter - Vitamins and supplements - Anything from herbalist or health store - Herbs - Teas - Traditions remedies
Medications information - Name - Dosage form - Dose - Schedule - Last dose taken - Be specific about prn medications use frequency - Ask about recently started medications, or dosage changes	**Use multiple sources of information** - Medication labels - Family - Community pharmacy - Family physician - If applicable, other health practitioners (e.g. naturopathic doctors)
Remember - Vague responses could be signs of non-compliance - Encourage patient to ask questions - Ask if patient is willing to bring the medications - Suggest the use of a medication wallet card - Offer a medication wallet card to the patient - Be specific about allergies (e.g. symptoms, causes, triggers, severity…)	**Type of questions to ask** - Open-ended questions - Yes/No questions when appropriate - Non-biased questions - No leading questions - Avoid medical jargon **Examples:** Did the doctor change the dose or stop any of your medications recently? How do you take this medication? Have you spent any days in the hospital for the past year? What are your concerns regarding your medications?

OSPE – Interactive Stations

.

Interactive Station #1 (Pharmacy Technician – Standardized Physician Interaction)

Your (Candidate) instructions:

Case description:

You are a pharmacy technician in a hospital pharmacy. Dr. Ali is waiting in the pharmacy to give you a new prescription for his patient Linda Thomas. Linda is suffering from headaches. You are expected to review the prescription below and answer as you would in practice.

Patient profile

Name: Linda Thomas
Gender: Female
Age: 27 years old
Medical History: Migraine headaches– recently diagnosed
Allergies: None
Current Medications (Rx & nRx): 1 Materna multivitamin daily, Maalox prn
Social/lifestyle: Non-smoker, no alcohol intake, physically active – gentle yoga 3 times a week

Station references: Compendium of Pharmaceuticals and Specialties (CPS)

This station must be completed in <u>6 minutes</u>

Prescription

Sunny Hospital
200 High Road
Rainy City
888-9970

For: Linda Thomas
Address: 88-4th Avenue

Correct date

Ergotamine
2 mg at onset of headache then 1 mg q1h prn x 3 doses

L. Ali

_____ Assume signature is correct
L. Ali M.D.

Standardized physician's introduction and questions

If asked, the physician will provide the following additional information:

Lynda had a baby girl 5 months ago and she is breastfeeding.

Important Note: The use of Materna (refer to profile) must prompt this investigation on your behalf. If you fail to ask, this key information will not be provided.

"Hi, I am Dr. Ali. I have a new prescription for my patient Linda Thomas."

If the candidate refers the physician to the pharmacist without identifying the problem, the standardized physician will ask:

"Is there a problem? What is wrong with the prescription?"

If the candidate says to avoid the medication without explaining, the standardized physician will ask:

"Could you explain why?"

STATION REVIEW FORM

<u>Write notes, answers, interview and counselling to show how you would solve this case</u>

Interactive Station #1 - Solution

Primary goals:

- Determine and confirm that the patient is a new mom who is breastfeeding.
- Identify and explain that ergotamine could suppress lactation.
- Explain that ergotamine could have adverse effects on the child as well since it is excreted in breast milk.
- Refer Dr. Ali to the pharmacist to discuss further.

The candidate is expected to:

Determine and confirm that the patient is breast feeding by interacting with Dr. Ali. Identify that the newly prescribed drug (ergotamine) could suppress lactation. Ergotamine is also excreted in breast milk which can potentially have adverse effects on the child.

Refer Dr. Ali to the pharmacist to determine the most appropriate treatment.

OSPE PERFORMANCE EVALUATION FORM

Communication skills (circle one)

4. Appropriate
3. Appropriate/Marginal
2. Poor/Marginal
1. Poor

Comments

```



```

Outcome (circle one)

4. Problem solved
3. Problem marginally solved
2. Problem not solved
1. Problem not identified

Comments

```



```

Performance (circle one)

4. Meets expectations
3. Meets expectations marginally
2. Does not meet expectations
1. Unacceptable

<u>Comments</u>

<table>
<tr><td></td></tr>
</table>

| Information inaccuracy | Yes | No |

| Risk to patient's safety | Yes | No |

Overall Mark

PASS   **FAIL**

Interactive Station #2 (Pharmacy Technician – Standardized Physician Interaction)

Your (Candidate) instructions:

Case description:

You are a pharmacy technician in a hospital pharmacy. Dr. Kim is waiting in the pharmacy to give you a new prescription for her patient Paul Sam for the management of diabetes.

Station references: Compendium of Pharmaceuticals and Specialties (CPS)

This station must be completed in 6 minutes

Patient profile

Name: Paul Sam
Gender: Male
Age: 57 years old
Medical History: COPD, one episode of lactic acidosis 7 months ago, hyperlipidemia, prediabetes– recently diagnosed
Allergies: None
Current Medications (Rx & nRx): Salbutamol 2 puffs tid prn, tiotropium 18 ug inhaled daily, atorvastatin 40 mg daily
Social/lifestyle: Non-smoker, no alcohol intake, he has been on low fat diet since his hyperlipidemia diagnosis, physically active – 4 times a week

Prescription

Honeydew Clinic
77 Spring Street
Canada City
999-7777

For: Paul Sam
Address: 4555-10th Avenue

Correct date

Metformin
100 mg divided bid x 3 months

R. Kim

_____ Assume signature is correct
R. Kim M.D.

Standardized physician's introduction and questions

"Hi, I am Dr. Kim. I have just written this new prescription for my patient Paul Sam."

If the candidate refers the physician to the pharmacist without identifying the problem, the standardized physician will ask:

"Is there a problem? What is wrong with the prescription?"

If the candidate says to avoid the medication without explaining, the standardized physician will ask:

"Could you explain why?"

STATION REVIEW FORM

Write notes, answers, interview and counselling to show how you would solve this case

Interactive Station #2 - Solution

<u>Primary goal</u>:

- Identify and confirm the patient's history of lactic acidosis
- Determine and explain that metformin is contraindicated in patients with history of lactic acidosis
- Refer Dr. Kim to the pharmacist to determine an appropriate treatment option

The candidate is expected to:

- Identify and confirm the patient's history of lactic acidosis.
- Determine and explain that metformin is contraindicated in patients with history of lactic acidosis
- Explain that lactic acidosis is one of the side effects of metformin therefore it should not be used in patients with history of lactic acidosis
- Refer Dr. Kim to the pharmacist to help determine the most appropriate treatment.

OSPE PERFORMANCE EVALUATION FORM

Communication skills (circle one)

4. Appropriate
3. Appropriate/Marginal
2. Poor/Marginal
1. Poor

Comments

```



```

Outcome (circle one)

4. Problem solved
3. Problem marginally solved
2. Problem not solved
1. Problem not identified

Comments

```



```

Performance (circle one)

4. Meets expectations
3. Meets expectations marginally
2. Does not meet expectations
1. Unacceptable

<u>Comments</u>

Information inaccuracy   Yes   No

Risk to patient's safety   Yes   No

Overall Mark

PASS   **FAIL**

Interactive Station #3 (Pharmacy Technician – Standardized Patient Interaction): Sunburn

Your (Candidate) instructions

Case description

You are a pharmacy technician in a community pharmacy. A 34-year-old female with severe erythema and peeling of her face, shoulders, and arms is visiting the pharmacy to seek your advice on how to manage her condition. She has spent most of the previous day at an outdoor farmers' market. She stated that this was the worst sunburn she had ever experienced. Provide your assistance as you would in practice.

This station must be completed in <u>6 minutes</u>

Station reference

Compendium of Pharmaceuticals and Specialties (CPS)

Patient profile

Patient Name: Anita Singh
Gender: Female
Age: 34 years old
Allergies: Seasonal
Medical History: Rheumatoid arthritis
Current medications (Rx & nRx): Methotrexate 15 mg po q week – dispensed 3 weeks ago,
Other: Advil prn for headaches, one daily multivitamin
Social/lifestyle: Non-smoker, no alcohol intake, physically active – visits the gym 5 times a week

Standardized patient's introduction and questions

"Hi, I am Anita. I have very bad sunburn. I was at the farmers' market yesterday. Could you tell me what kind of product will help? I have never had anything like that."

STATION REVIEW FORM

<u>Write notes, answers, interview and counselling to show how you would solve this case</u>

Interactive Station #3 - Solution

Primary goals:

- Confirm patient's identity
- Confirm that the patient is on methotrexate
- Determine that the patient is suffering from methotrexate-induced photosensitivity. Her symptoms, exposure to methotrexate and lack of history of similar reaction are likely indicative of phototoxic reaction. The onset of the reaction (within 24 hrs) is also consistent with phototoxicity.
- Discuss non-drug strategies to minimize photosensitivity (see below)
- Identify and explain that NSAIDs (Advil) increase the levels of methotrexate which could worsen her photosensitivity.
- Refer her to the pharmacist to discuss further

The candidate is expected to:

Discuss non drug strategies to minimize the risk of photosensitive reactions:

- Avoid direct UV exposure from natural sunlight as well as tanning beds. Especially avoid the sun between 10 a.m. and 3 p.m.

- Wear sun-protective clothing when going outdoors. If possible, wear shirts with high collars and long sleeves, pants or a long skirt, socks and shoes, a wide-brimmed hat, and sunglasses.

- Use a UV-A and UV-B combination sunscreen with at least SPF 15.

- Mild reactions could be managed by applying cool wet dressings.

Refer the patient to the pharmacist to help determine the most appropriate course of action.

<u>Further learning:</u>

Photosensitivity reactions can be classified into two categories:

Phototoxic reactions. Ultraviolet (UV) light activates the photosensitizing drug to emit energy that may damage adjacent skin tissue resulting in an intensified sunburn with skin peeling. Phototoxicity is characterized by a rapid onset of erythema, pain, prickling, or burning sensation of areas exposed to the sun, with peak symptoms occurring 12-24 hours after the initial exposure. The hallmark of this reaction is the appearance of a sunburn-like reaction on areas of skin with the greatest exposure to sunlight. These reactions do not involve the immune system; therefore, prior exposure or sensitization to a drug is not necessary for this reaction to occur.
Factors influencing the intensity and incidence of drug-induced phototoxicity include:
- The concentration, absorption, and pharmacokinetics of the drug.
- The dose of sunlight (duration of exposure and spectrum of sunlight).

Photoallergic reactions. Drug induced photoallergy is less common than phototoxicity and requires prolonged or prior exposure to the photosensitizing drug. As the name suggests, this type of reaction is immune mediated. UV light reacts with the drug to produce an immunogenic hapten resulting in cell mediated immune response resulting in a skin reaction. Photoallergic reactions are not dose dependent and are characterized by urticaria (called solar hives) with eczema-like dermatitis and erythema. Light exposed areas on the skin are the predominant location of the reaction. These eruptions usually disappear spontaneously upon removal of the offending drug.

OSPE PERFORMANCE EVALUATION FORM

Communication skills (circle one)

4. Appropriate
3. Appropriate/Marginal
2. Poor/Marginal
1. Poor

Comments

```
┌──────────────────────────────────────────────────┐
│                                                    │
│                                                    │
│                                                    │
│                                                    │
│                                                    │
└──────────────────────────────────────────────────┘
```

Outcome (circle one)

4. Problem solved
3. Problem marginally solved
2. Problem not solved
1. Problem not identified

Comments

```
┌──────────────────────────────────────────────────┐
│                                                    │
│                                                    │
│                                                    │
│                                                    │
│                                                    │
└──────────────────────────────────────────────────┘
```

Performance (circle one)

4. Meets expectations
3. Meets expectations marginally
2. Does not meet expectations
1. Unacceptable

Comments

Information inaccuracy   Yes   No

Risk to patient's safety   Yes   No

Overall Mark

PASS   **FAIL**

Interactive Station #4 (Pharmacy Technician – Standardized Pharmacy Technician Interaction): Ethics

<u>Case description</u>:

Nicole Dylan is your longtime colleague. You are both experienced pharmacy technicians. You have been good friends for almost twelve years; she is like your big sister. Nicole told you confidentially that she has been making lot of mistakes lately, she is being very forgetful. Nicole is turning 58 in 2 months. She mentioned that her recent physical exam showed that she is in good health. She thinks her forgetfulness is simply showing her age. She explains that her work is becoming very stressful because she is constantly worried about harming someone due to her forgetfulness. Answer as you would in practice.

STATION REVIEW FORM

Write notes, answers, interview and counselling to show how you would solve this case

Interactive Station #4 - Solution

The candidate is expected:

First, comfort and provide support to Nicole. Reassure that she can always count on your support and friendship.

Assure she is not alone. Many aging professionals are feeling the impact of their age on the workplace. The Canadian workforce is aging.

Remind Nicole that the safety of patients must be a priority.

Encourage her to discuss the matter openly with the pharmacy manager. The manager could offer a different work assignment or another workable solution

Discuss the situation with the manager if Nicole decides **not to disclose** her shortcomings to the manager. Failure to do that will be against the principle of non-maleficence. A prompt resolution of the issue will be also in the best interest of Nicole because a fatal mistake has major consequences. Nicole's lack of cooperation could jeopardize the safety of patients.

OSPE PERFORMANCE EVALUATION FORM

Communication skills (circle one)

4. Appropriate
3. Appropriate/Marginal
2. Poor/Marginal
1. Poor

Comments

Outcome (circle one)

4. Problem solved
3. Problem marginally solved
2. Problem not solved
1. Problem not identified

Comments

Performance (circle one)

4. Meets expectations
3. Meets expectations marginally
2. Does not meet expectations
1. Unacceptable

<u>Comments</u>

Information inaccuracy   Yes   No

Risk to patient's safety   Yes   No

Overall Mark

PASS   **FAIL**

Interactive Station #5 (Pharmacy Technician – Standardized Patient Interaction): Headaches

Your (Candidate) instructions

<u>Case description</u>:

You are pharmacy technician in a community pharmacy. A patient is visiting your pharmacy complaining about the lack of effectiveness of her headaches medication. She has been using Imitrex for the past 2 months. Unfortunately, her condition is not well controlled despite the use of the maximum dose of 200 mg daily for at least 3 days weekly. She has recently noticed that her condition has worsened resulting in recurrent headaches. She is wondering if adding Tylenol to her current medication regimen would improve her condition. Provide your assistance as you would in practice.

This station must be completed in <u>6 minutes</u>

<u>Station materials and references</u>:

Compendium of Pharmaceuticals and Specialties (CPS)
Compendium of Products for Minor Ailments

Patient profile

Patient Name: June Smith
Gender: Female
Age: 35 years old
Allergies: None known
Medical History: Migraine headaches, GERD - controlled
Current medications (Rx & nRx): Imitrex 200 mg daily, one multivitamin daily
Social/lifestyle: Secondary school teacher, non-smoker, no alcohol use, physically inactive – enjoys running 3 times weekly

Standardized patient's introduction and questions

"Hi, I am June Smith. I have been using a medication for headaches for the past two months. It doesn't seem to work. I am using it at least 3 days per week. I would like to have your advice on adding Tylenol. Do you think I will finally feel better? How much Tylenol should I take?"

If not addressed by the candidate after 4 1/2 minutes, the standardized patient will ask the following question:

"Do you know why my headaches have worsened?

If the candidate refers the patient to the pharmacist without identifying the problem, the patient will ask:

"Could you explain why? What is wrong with my medication?"

STATION REVIEW FORM

Write notes, answers, interview and counselling to show how you would solve this case

Interactive Station #5 - Solution

<u>Primary goals</u>:

- Confirm patient's identity
- Confirm that the patient is on Imitrex
- Confirm that the patient needs Imitrex
- Determine that the patient is suffering from medication-overuse headache.
- Explain that Imitrex should not be use more than 10 days a month.
- Refer the patient to the pharmacist to determine the best course of action

The candidate is expected to:

Identify that the patient is suffering from rebound or medication overuse headaches.

Explain that Imitrex should not be use more than 10 days a month.

Recommend having a headache diary which would help monitor the effectiveness of treatment.

Discuss the following headache management strategies: avoid triggers, apply ice, rest in a dark noise-free room and relaxation

Refer the patient to the pharmacist to help determine the most appropriate course of action.

OSPE PERFORMANCE EVALUATION FORM

Communication skills (circle one)

4. Appropriate
3. Appropriate/Marginal
2. Poor/Marginal
1. Poor

Comments

```



```

Outcome (circle one)

4. Problem solved
3. Problem marginally solved
2. Problem not solved
1. Problem not identified

Comments

```



```

Performance (circle one)

4. Meets expectations
3. Meets expectations marginally
2. Does not meet expectations
1. Unacceptable

Comments

```


```

Information inaccuracy	Yes	No
Risk to patient's safety	Yes	No

Overall Mark

PASS   **FAIL**

Interactive Station #6 (Pharmacist – Standardized Patient Interaction): Proper use of an inhaler

Your (Candidate) instructions

Case description:

You are pharmacy technician in a community pharmacy. Mr. Young has been a long-time smoker. After few months of recurrent cough, he has been diagnosed with congestive obstructive pulmonary disease (COPD). He is visiting your pharmacy with a new prescription for Atroven HFA (Ipratropium). He is expecting to learn how to properly use his puffer. Provide your assistance as you would in practice.

This station must be completed in 6 minutes

Station materials and references:

Compendium of Pharmaceuticals and Specialties (CPS)
Compendium of Products for Minor Ailments
Atroven HFA

Patient profile

Patient Name: Peter Young
Gender: Male
Age: 69 years old
Allergies: None
Medical History: Glaucoma
Current medications (Rx & nRx): Dorzolamide 1 drop Q8, 1 daily multivitamin, Tylenol for occasional back pain
New prescription: Atroven HFA 2 puffs Q6 daily
Social/lifestyle: Retired, lives alone with family support, stopped smoking 3 years ago, no alcohol intake, enjoys swimming – 3 times weekly

Standardized patient's introduction and questions

"Hi, I just got this new prescription from my doctor. It is my first time taking this medication and I am not sure how to use it properly. Could you show me how to use it?"

STATION REVIEW FORM

Write notes, answers, interview and counselling to show how you would solve this case

Interactive Station #6 - Solution

Primary goals:

- Confirm patient's identity
- Confirm that the patient needs Atroven HFA
- Explain the benefits of using Atroven HFA
- Educate the patient on how to use the inhaler
- Determine that ipratropium could adversely affect the patient's glaucoma
- Refer the patient to the pharmacist to further discuss how ipratropium could affect glaucoma

The candidate is expected to:

Discuss the drug schedule with the patient. 2 puffs every 6 hours.

Explain how to use the Metered Dose Inhaler (MDI):
- Atroven HFA is a solution aerosol that does not require shaking
- Remove the cap
- Prime with 2 test sprays before first use. If the inhaler has not been used for more than 3 days, prime again by releasing 2 test sprays into the air away from the face.
- Breathe out, away from your inhaler
- Bring the inhaler to your mouth. Place it in your mouth between your teeth and close your mouth around it.
- Start to breathe in slowly. Press the top of your inhaler once and keep breathing in slowly until you have taken a full breath.
- Remove the inhaler from your mouth, and hold your breath for about 10 seconds, then breathe out.
- Wait 30s to 1 min before another puff. Repeat steps 3 to 6.
- Store the MDI at room temperature. If it gets cold, warm it using only your hands. When using a new MDI, write the start date on the canister. Check the expiry date on the MDI before use.
- Avoid contact with eyes to help minimize adverse effect on eye such as worsening of glaucoma. Advise to seek medical help immediately if vision changes
- Do not exceed 12 inhalations in 24 hours.
- The minimum interval between doses should not be less than 4 hours.

Discuss non-pharmacologic strategies:
- Avoid exposure to air pollution
- Physical activity helps improve symptoms
- Refer the patient to the pharmacist to discuss how ipratropium could affect glaucoma. Glaucoma monitoring maybe initiated.

OSPE PERFORMANCE EVALUATION FORM

Communication skills (circle one)

4. Appropriate
3. Appropriate/Marginal
2. Poor/Marginal
1. Poor

Comments

```


```

Outcome (circle one)

4. Problem solved
3. Problem marginally solved
2. Problem not solved
1. Problem not identified

Comments

```


```

Performance (circle one)

4. Meets expectations
3. Meets expectations marginally
2. Does not meet expectations
1. Unacceptable

<u>Comments</u>

Information inaccuracy	Yes	No
Risk to patient's safety	Yes	No

Overall Mark

PASS   **FAIL**

Interactive Station #7 (Pharmacy Technician– Standardized Patient Interaction): Omega-3 oil supplement

Your (Candidate) instructions

Case description:

You are a pharmacy technician in a community pharmacy. An elderly patient is visiting the pharmacy to seek your assistance to select an omega 3 oil supplement. A friend told him that omega-3 has several health benefits but he is still hesitant to take the product. He seems to be overwhelmed by the choices available. Provide your assistance as you would in practice.

This station must be completed in <u>6 minutes</u>

Station materials and references:

Natural Medicines Comprehensive Database
Cod fish oil – Omega-3, Vitamin A &Vitamin D bottle
Omega-3 EPA DHA 500 mg bottle

Patient profile

Patient Name: Joe Smith
Gender: Male
Age: 49 years old
Allergies: None
Medical History: Borderline type 2 diabetes managed with diet
Current medications (Rx & nRx): None
Other: Tylenol prn, one daily multivitamin
Social/lifestyle: Non-smoker, no alcohol intake, physically active – visits the gym 5 times a week

Standardized patient's introduction and questions

"Hi, could you tell me which one of these two products is best (refer to station materials)? A friend told me that omega-3 has many health benefits. I haven't used it yet. I am not sure how much will be enough. Could you help me with that?"

If the candidate refers the patient to the pharmacist without identifying the problem, the standardized patient will ask:

"Could you explain why?"

If the candidate says to avoid one of the products without explaining, the standardized patient will ask:

"Could you explain why?"

If not addressed by the candidate after 4 1/2 minutes, the standardized patient will ask the following:

"How many capsules should I take daily?"

STATION REVIEW FORM

<u>Write notes, answers, interview and counselling to show how you would solve this case</u>

Interactive Station #7 - Solution

<u>Primary goals</u>:

- Patient education. Discuss the difference between the two omega-3 oil supplements in the station.
- Identify that Omega-3 EPA DHA 500 mg would be a better option

The candidate is expected to explain that:

Fish liver oils, such as cod liver oil, are not the same as fish oil. Fish liver oils contain vitamins A and D as well as omega-3 fatty acids. Both of these vitamins can be unsafe in large doses. Therefore, omega-3 EPA DHA 500 mg would be preferred.

The standard recommended daily intake of omega-3 is 1000 mg (EPA + DHA). Therefore, the patient will need 2 capsules daily.

Discuss the health benefits of omega-3. Omega-3 fats have been shown to help prevent heart disease and stroke, help control lupus, eczema, and rheumatoid arthritis, and may play protective roles in cancer, inflammation, sleep and brain function.

Discuss that salmon is a good source of omega-3.

Salmon (wild)	6.0 oz	1,774 mg of Omega-3
Salmon (farmed)	6.0 oz	4,504 mg of Omega-3

Ask the patient if he would like to talk to the pharmacist.

<u>Further learning</u>:

Dosing for fish oil supplements should be based on the amount of EPA (Eicosapentaenoic Acid) and DHA (Docosahexaenoic Acid), not on the total amount of fish oil. Supplements have different amounts of EPA and DHA. The recommended dose is 1000 mg daily of EPA and DHA combined.

OSPE PERFORMANCE EVALUATION FORM

Communication skills (circle one)

4. Appropriate
3. Appropriate/Marginal
2. Poor/Marginal
1. Poor

Comments

```
┌──────────────────────────────────────────────────┐
│                                                    │
│                                                    │
│                                                    │
│                                                    │
│                                                    │
│                                                    │
└──────────────────────────────────────────────────┘
```

Outcome (circle one)

4. Problem solved
3. Problem marginally solved
2. Problem not solved
1. Problem not identified

Comments

```
┌──────────────────────────────────────────────────┐
│                                                    │
│                                                    │
│                                                    │
│                                                    │
│                                                    │
│                                                    │
└──────────────────────────────────────────────────┘
```

Performance (circle one)

4. Meets expectations
3. Meets expectations marginally
2. Does not meet expectations
1. Unacceptable

<u>Comments</u>

Information inaccuracy   Yes   No

Risk to patient's safety   Yes   No

Overall Mark

PASS   **FAIL**

Interactive Station #8 (Pharmacy Technician– Standardized Patient Interaction): Antacid

Your (Candidate) instructions

Case description:

You are a pharmacy technician in a community pharmacy. A female patient is seeking your assistance to select an antacid to manage occasional heartburn. She had experienced few episodes of diarrhea with her antacid; unfortunately, she does not recall which antacid she had used. She seems to be overwhelmed by the different types of antacids available.

This station must be completed in 6 minutes

Station materials and references:

Compendium of Products for Minor Ailments

OTC antacids:
Alka Seltzer
Maalox liquid
Milk of Magnesia
Pepto-Bismol

Patient profile

Patient Name: Marie John
Gender: Female
Age: 67 years old
Allergies: Aspirin
Medical History: Hypertension, postherpetic neuralgia
Current medications (Rx & nRx): Hydrochlorothiazide 25 mg once a day, Gabapentin 300 mg tid, Tylenol prn for headaches
Social/lifestyle: Non-smoker, No alcohol consumption, physically active – daily 35 minutes walk

Standardized patient's introduction and questions

"Hi, could you tell me which of these products is best for my heartburns? I had diarrhea with one of them, but I don't remember which one. I am just looking for something that works for me. Could you help me?"

4 OTC medications are available in the station.

If not addressed by the candidate after 41/2 minutes, the standardized patient should ask:

"Can I use it with my other medications?"

"Should I expect to have diarrhea again?"

STATION REVIEW FORM

<u>Write notes, answers, interview and counselling to show how you would solve this case</u>

Interactive Station #8 - Solution

<u>Primary goals:</u>

- Confirm patient's identity
- Confirm that the patient needs antacid
- Identify the antacid linked to diarrhea (Mg containing product such as Milk of Magnesia)
- Determine that Maalox contains both Mg (diarrhea inducer) and Alu (constipation inducer) which provides a good balance; the likelihood of diarrhea and constipation are both minimized.
- Advise to avoid Na containing products such as Alka Seltzer due to possible adverse effect on hypertension
- Advise to avoid aspirin containing Pepto-Bismol due to her aspirin allergy
- Identify the interaction between gabapentin and antacid
- Refer the patient to the pharmacist to discuss further

The candidate is expected to:

Explain why Alka Seltzer and Milk of Magnesia and Pepto-Bismol should be avoided

Discuss the interaction between antacid and gabapentin; antacids reduce the absorption of gabapentin.

Congratulate and encourage the patient to continue staying active. Discuss briefly the benefits of physical activity in hypertensive patients. Recall other non-pharmacologic strategies in the management of hypertension such as weight loss and healthy diet.

Recommend the application of a washcloth dipped in cool water to help reduce shingles pain and dry the blisters. Suggest stress reduction strategies such as relaxation techniques to help manage the pain. In addition, explain that good body hygiene helps reduce secondary bacterial infections.

Refer the patient to the pharmacist to discuss how to manage gabapentin-antacid interaction.

<u>Further learning:</u>
Take Maalox at least 2 hours before taking gabapentin to minimize the interaction

OSPE PERFORMANCE EVALUATION FORM

Communication skills (circle one)

4. Appropriate
3. Appropriate/Marginal
2. Poor/Marginal
1. Poor

Comments

```



```

Outcome (circle one)

4. Problem solved
3. Problem marginally solved
2. Problem not solved
1. Problem not identified

Comments

```



```

Performance (circle one)

4. Meets expectations
3. Meets expectations marginally
2. Does not meet expectations
1. Unacceptable

Comments

Information inaccuracy   Yes   No

Risk to patient's safety   Yes   No

Overall Mark

PASS   **FAIL**

Interactive Station #9 (Pharmacy Technician– Standardized Patient Interaction): Smoking cessation

Your (Candidate) instructions

<u>Case description:</u>

You are a pharmacy technician in a community pharmacy. A male patient is visiting the pharmacy to seek your assistance regarding the use of nicotine gum to help him quit smoking. Following an earlier counseling session, the pharmacist has recommended 4 mg gum; Derek is a heavy smoker. His previous attempts without stop smoking aid have not been successful. He is once again fully committed and very optimistic about the outcome. Provide your assistance as you would in practice.

This station must be completed in <u>6 minutes</u>

<u>Station materials and references:</u>

Compendium of Products for Minor Ailments
A pack of 4 mg Nicotine Gum

Patient profile

Patient Name: Derek Ming
Gender: Male
Age: 32 years old
Allergies: Seasonal allergies
Medical History: None
Current medications (Rx & nRx): None
Social/lifestyle: Fitness instructor, smoker for 10 years – more than 1 and 1/2 pack daily, moderate alcohol intake – 3 drinks weekly.

Standardized patient's introduction and questions

"Hi, I just talked to the pharmacist and he has recommended the 4 mg gum. Could you explain how I should use it? I have not been successful quitting without medication."

Note: The standardized patient shows some signs of optimism and excitement about stop smoking.

He is planning to stop smoking in 3 days.

STATION REVIEW FORM

<u>Write notes, answers, interview and counselling to show how you would solve this case</u>

Interactive Station #9 - Solution

Primary goals:

- Confirm patient's identity
- Confirm that the patient needs nicotine gum
- Explain the benefits of using nicotine gum to stop smoking
- Educate the patient on the use of nicotine gum

The candidate is expected to:

Reassure the patient that previous failures do not prevent future success.

Advise the following regimen for 4 mg gum:

- 10 to 12 pieces/day initially to max of 20 pieces for 8 to 12 weeks then reduce by 1 piece daily each week as withdrawal symptoms allow.
- Then gradually decrease the total number of pieces used per day.
- Gradually replace 4 mg gum with 2 mg gum.
- Gradual reduction of chewing time from 30 minutes to 10 to 15 minutes is also a helpful dose reduction strategy.

Explain that nicotine gum should be chewed slowly until he can taste the nicotine or feel a slight tingling in his mouth. Then stop chewing and place the gum between the cheek and gum. When the tingling is almost gone (usually within 1 minute), start chewing again. Repeat for about 30 minutes. Do not chew nicotine gum too fast, do not chew more than one piece of gum at a time, and do not chew one piece too soon after another. He should plan to stop using the gum when his craving for nicotine is satisfied by one or two pieces of gum per day.

Avoid smoking. Explain that smoking while using nicotine gum may cause the buildup of nicotine to toxic levels.

Recommend follow-up to monitor progress and provide encouragement.

OSPE PERFORMANCE EVALUATION FORM

Communication skills (circle one)

4. Appropriate
3. Appropriate/Marginal
2. Poor/Marginal
1. Poor

Comments

Outcome (circle one)

4. Problem solved
3. Problem marginally solved
2. Problem not solved
1. Problem not identified

Comments

Performance (circle one)

4. Meets expectations
3. Meets expectations marginally
2. Does not meet expectations
1. Unacceptable

<u>Comments</u>

Information inaccuracy   Yes   No

Risk to patient's safety   Yes   No

Overall Mark

PASS   **FAIL**

Interactive Station #10 (Pharmacy Technician– Standardized Patient Interaction): Application of nasal spray

Your (Candidate) instructions

Case description:

You are a pharmacy technician in a community pharmacy. A young male patient is seeking your advice on the use of a non-prescription nasal spray he has just purchased. He has a cold and has been dealing with nasal congestion for about a day. He would like also to know how many sprays will be needed and for how long he can use it. Provide your assistance as you would in practice.

Station materials and references:

Compendium of Products for Minor Ailments
Drixoral Nasal Spray (oxymetazoline nasal spray)

This station must be completed in 6 minutes

There is no patient's profile in this station. If asked, the standardized patient will provide the following information:

Patient Name: Sam Michael
Age: 20 years old
Allergies: None
Medical History: None
Current medications (Rx & nRx): None
Social/lifestyle: College student, non-smoker, no alcohol intake, plays volleyball at least 3 times a week

Standardized patient's introduction and questions

"Hi, I just got this nasal spray. I have been dealing with stuffy nose for about a day, I have a cold. Could you show me how to use it properly? How many sprays do I need?"

If not addressed by the candidate after 41/2 minutes, the standardized patient will ask:

"How many sprays do I need?"

"For how long I can use it?"

STATION REVIEW FORM

<u>Write notes, answers, interview and counselling to show how you would solve this case</u>

Interactive Station #10 - Solution

Primary goal:

- Confirm patient's identity
- Confirm that the patient needs nasal decongestant
- Explain the benefits of Drixoral
- Demonstration of the use of Drixoral Nasal Spray (oxymetazoline nasal spray)
- Make recommendations according to the package instructions

The candidate is expected to:

Demonstrate and explain the proper use of nasal spray:

- Wash your hands thoroughly with soap and water
- Blow your nose gently before using the spray
- Remove the cap and gently insert the bottle tip into one nostril. Press the other nostril with one finger.
- Keep your head upright. Squeeze the bottle to release the product, and then sniff deeply.
- Repeat in the other nostril
- Wipe clean the nozzle
- Store at room temperature

Recommend according to the package instructions: 2 to 3 sprays in each nostril every 10 to 12 hours and not to use the spray for more than 3 days to prevent rebound congestion (worsening of congestion)

Discuss non-drug strategies:

- Use gentle saline nasal sprays.
- Increase the humidity in the air with a vaporizer or humidifier.
- Drink extra fluids. Hot tea, broth, or chicken soup.

OSPE PERFORMANCE EVALUATION FORM

Communication skills (circle one)

4. Appropriate
3. Appropriate/Marginal
2. Poor/Marginal
1. Poor

Comments

```



```

Outcome (circle one)

4. Problem solved
3. Problem marginally solved
2. Problem not solved
1. Problem not identified

Comments

```



```

Performance (circle one)

4. Meets expectations
3. Meets expectations marginally
2. Does not meet expectations
1. Unacceptable

Comments

Information inaccuracy   Yes   No

Risk to patient's safety   Yes   No

Overall Mark

PASS   **FAIL**

OSPE Non-Interactive Stations

Non-interactive Station #1: Dispensed Prescriptions Check

Candidate's instructions:

Identify any problem(s) related to the dispensed **product** and **label**, **if any**, that must be addressed prior to releasing the product. Mark **all** identified problem(s) on the answer form by filling the circle(s). You have a total of **4 prescriptions** in this station.

This station must be completed in 6 minutes

Written Rx 1

Rx 1
Patient Name: Miranda Smith
Address: 35 Hill Street

Correct date

Gleevec
800 mg divided bid for leukemia for 90 days

K. Junior

_____ Assume signature is correct
K. Junior M.D.

Dispensed Rx 1 label

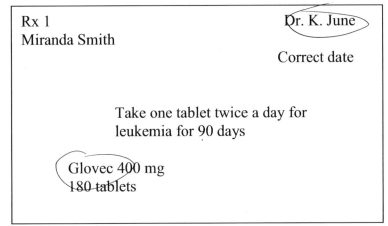

Rx 1
Miranda Smith

Dr. K. June

Correct date

Take one tablet twice a day for
leukemia for 90 days

Glovec 400 mg
180 tablets

Rx1: Dispensed Product

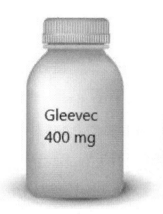

Gleevec
400 mg

Written Rx 2

Rx 2
Patient Name: Heather Moon
Address: 34C Street

                                                        Correct date

   Fluconazole
   150 mg po x 1 dose for vaginal candidiasis

        N. Smith
_____   Assume signature is correct
        N. Smith M.D.

Dispensed Rx 2 label

Rx 2   Dr. N. Smith
Heather Moon
                                        Correct date

             Take three tablets once
             for vaginal candidiasis

      Fluconazole 50 mg

      3 tablets

Rx2: Dispensed Product

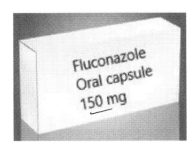

Fluconazole
Oral capsule
150 mg

Written Rx 3

Rx 3
Patient Name: Fanny May
Address: 2123 Street

Correct date

Mirtazapine
15 mg tab once a day x 8 weeks

F. Tom

_____ Assume signature is correct
F. Tom M.D.

Dispensed Rx 3 label

Rx 3   Dr. P. Tom
Fanny Pete

Correct date

Take one tablet once a day
for eight weeks

Mirtazapine 15 mg

56 tablets

Rx3: Dispensed Product

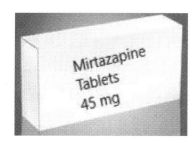

Written Rx 4

Rx 4
Patient Name: Lynn Ryan
Address: 311 Summer Street

Correct date

Norfloxacin
400 mg po bid 1 h ac x 3 days

K. Lam

_____   Assume signature is correct
K. Lam M.D.

Dispensed Rx 4 label

Rx 4   Dr. K. Liam
Lynn<u>a</u> Ryan

Correct date

Take one tablet twice a day one hour
after a m<u>ea</u>l for three days

Norfloxacin 400 mg

6 tablets

Rx4: Dispensed Product

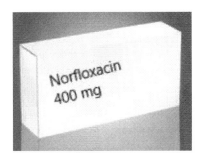

Answer Form #1

Rx1 Dispensed product related problems (refer to enclosed images)	Rx1 Label related problems
O Drug ID O Drug dosage form O Drug strength O Drug packaging ⊘ No product problem	⊘ Physician name O Patient name ⊘ Drug name O Drug quantity O Drug strength O Drug dosage form O Directions of use O No label problem
Rx2 Dispensed product related problems (refer to enclosed images)	Rx2 Label related problems (refer to enclosed Rx label)
O Drug ID O Drug dosage form ⊘ Drug strength O Drug packaging O No product problem	O Physician name O Patient name O Drug name O Drug quantity ⊘ Drug strength O Drug dosage form O Directions of use ⊘ No label problem
Rx3 Dispensed product related problems (refer to enclosed images)	Rx3 Label related problems (refer to enclosed Rx label)
O Drug ID O Drug dosage form ⊘ Drug strength O Drug packaging O No product problem	O Physician name ⊘ Patient name O Drug name O Drug quantity O Drug strength O Drug dosage form O Directions of use

	O No label problem
Rx4 Dispensed product related problems (refer to enclosed images)	Rx4 Label related problems (refer to enclosed Rx label)
<ul><li>O Drug ID</li><li>O Drug dosage form</li><li>O Drug strength</li><li>O Drug packaging</li><li>O No product problem</li></ul>	<ul><li>O Physician name</li><li>⊘ Patient name</li><li>O Drug name</li><li>O Drug quantity</li><li>O Drug strength</li><li>O Drug dosage form</li><li>⊘ Directions of use (before meals – ac)</li><li>O No label problem</li></ul>

Answer Key #1

Rx1 Dispensed product related problems (refer to enclosed images)	**Rx1** Label related problems
○ Drug ID ○ Drug dosage form ○ Drug strength ○ Drug packaging ● **No product problem**	● **Physician name** ○ Patient name ● **Drug name** ○ Drug quantity ○ Drug strength ○ Drug dosage form ○ Directions of use ○ No label problem
Rx2 Dispensed product related problems (refer to enclosed images)	**Rx2** Label related problems (refer to enclosed Rx label)
○ Drug ID ○ Drug dosage form ● **Drug strength** ○ Drug packaging ○ No product problem	○ Physician name ○ Patient name ○ Drug name ○ Drug quantity ○ Drug strength ○ Drug dosage form ○ Directions of use ● **No label problem**
Rx3 Dispensed product related problems (refer to enclosed images)	**Rx3** Label related problems (refer to enclosed Rx label)
○ Drug ID ○ Drug dosage form ● **Drug strength** ○ Drug packaging ○ No product problem	● **Physician name** ● **Patient name** ○ Drug name ○ Drug quantity ○ Drug strength ○ Drug dosage form

	O Directions of use
	O No label problem
Rx4 Dispensed product related problems (refer to enclosed images)	**Rx4** Label related problems (refer to enclosed Rx label)
O Drug ID O Drug dosage form O Drug strength O Drug packaging ● **No product problem**	● **Physician name** ● **Patient name** O Drug name O Drug quantity O Drug strength O Drug dosage form ● **Directions of use (before meals – ac)** O No label problem

Non-interactive Station #2: Dispensed Prescriptions Check

Candidate's instructions:

Identify any problem(s) related to the dispensed **product** and **label**, **if any**, that must be corrected prior to releasing the product. Mark **all** identified problem(s) on the answer form by filling the circle(s). You have a total of **4 prescriptions** in this station.

<u>This station must be completed in 6 minutes</u>

Written Rx 1

Rx 1
Patient Name: Kim Park
Address: 30 Seaview Drive

Correct date

Neomycin 3.5 mg/g cream
Apply twice a day x 7 days to affected area

K. Gill
_____   Assume signature is correct
K. Gill M.D.

Dispensed Rx 1 label

Rx 1   Dr. K. Gill
Kim Park

Correct date

Apply twice daily for seven days to
affected area

Neomycin 3.5 mg/ml cream

Rx1: Dispensed Product

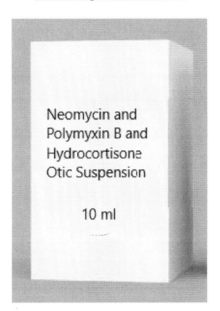

Neomycin and
Polymyxin B and
Hydrocortisone
Otic Suspension

10 ml

Written Rx 2

Rx 2
Patient Name: Timmy Hamed
Address: 22 Sunny Place

Correct date

Paliperidone ER
6 mg daily x 5 days, then 12 mg daily x 2 weeks

Y. Patrick

_____ Assume signature is correct
Y. Patrick M.D.

Dispensed Rx 2 label

Rx 2   Dr. Y. Patrick
                    Timmy Hamed
                                        Correct date

            Take two tablets once a day
            for five days then take fours tablets a day
            for fourteen days

        Paliperidone ER 3 mg

        66 tablets

<u>Rx2: Dispensed Product</u>

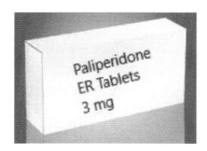

Written Rx 3

Rx 3
Patient Name: April Lee
Address: 21 Winter Blv

                                                    Correct date

        Medroxyprogesterone
        20 mg tid x 4 weeks

            A. Whyth
        _____   Assume signature is correct
            A. Whyth M.D.

Dispensed Rx 3 label

Rx 3   Dr. A. Whyth
April Lee

                                   Correct date

                Take two tablets three times a day
                for four weeks

           Medraprogesterone 10 mg

              168 tablets

Rx3: Dispensed Product

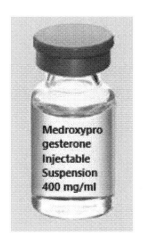

Written Rx 4

Rx 4
Patient Name: Andrea Fynn
Address: 34A Street

                                       Correct date

         Norethindrone 5mg
         10 mg on day 5 through day 25 of menstrual cycle for
         amenorrhea

          N. Smith

_____   Assume signature is correct
      N. Smith M.D.

Dispensed Rx 4 label

Rx 4   Dr. N. Smith
Andrea Fynn
                                                      Correct date

Take two tablets on day 5 through day 25 of
menstrual cycle for amenorrhea

Norethindrone 10 mg

40 tablets

Rx4: Dispensed Product

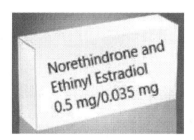

Answer Form #2

Rx1 Dispensed product related problems (refer to enclosed images)	Rx1 Label related problems
⊘ Drug ID ⊘ Drug dosage form ○ Drug strength ○ Drug packaging ○ No product problem	○ Physician name ○ Patient name ○ Drug name ○ Drug quantity ○ Drug strength ○ Drug dosage form ○ Directions of use ⊘ No label problem
Rx2 Dispensed product related problems (refer to enclosed images)	**Rx2 Label related problems (refer to enclosed Rx label)**
○ Drug ID ○ Drug dosage form ○ Drug strength ○ Drug packaging ⊘ No product problem	○ Physician name ○ Patient name ○ Drug name ○ Drug quantity ○ Drug strength ○ Drug dosage form ○ Directions of use ⊘ No label problem
Rx3 Dispensed product related problems (refer to enclosed images)	**Rx3 Label related problems (refer to enclosed Rx label)**
⊘ Drug ID ⊘ Drug dosage form ⊘ Drug strength ○ Drug packaging ○ No product problem	○ Physician name ○ Patient name ⊘ Drug name ○ Drug quantity ○ Drug strength ○ Drug dosage form ○ Directions of use

	O No label problem
Rx4 Dispensed product related problems (refer to enclosed images)	Rx4 Label related problems (refer to enclosed Rx label)
☑ Drug ID O Drug dosage form ☑ Drug strength O Drug packaging O No product problem	O Physician name O Patient name O Drug name O Drug quantity ☑ Drug strength O Drug dosage form O Directions of use (before meals – ac) O No label problem

Answer Key #2

Rx1 Dispensed product related problems (refer to enclosed images)	**Rx1** Label related problems
● **Drug ID (wrong product)** ● **Drug dosage form** ○ Drug strength ○ Drug packaging ○ No product problem	○ Physician name ○ Patient name ○ Drug name ○ Drug quantity ○ Drug strength ○ Drug dosage form ○ Directions of use ● **No label problem**
Rx2 Dispensed product related problems (refer to enclosed images)	**Rx2** Label related problems (refer to enclosed Rx label)
○ Drug ID ○ Drug dosage form ○ Drug strength ○ Drug packaging ● **No product problem**	○ Physician name ○ Patient name ○ Drug name ○ Drug quantity ○ Drug strength ○ Drug dosage form ○ Directions of use ● **No label problem**
Rx3 Dispensed product related problems (refer to enclosed images)	**Rx3** Label related problems (refer to enclosed Rx label)
○ Drug ID ● **Drug dosage form** ● **Drug strength** ○ Drug packaging ○ No product problem	○ Physician name ○ Patient name ● **Drug name** ○ Drug quantity ○ Drug strength ○ Drug dosage form ○ Directions of use ○ No label problem

Rx4 Dispensed product related problems (refer to enclosed images)	**Rx4** Label related problems (refer to enclosed Rx label)
● **Drug ID** ○ Drug dosage form ● **Drug strength** ○ Drug packaging ○ No product problem	○ Physician name ○ Patient name ● **Drug name** ○ Drug quantity ● **Drug strength (5 gm not 10 mg)** ○ Drug dosage form ○ Directions of use ○ No label problem

Non-interactive Station #3: Dispensed Prescriptions Check

Candidate's instructions:

Identify any problem(s) related to the dispensed **product** and **label**, **if any**, that must be corrected prior to releasing the product. Mark **all** identified problem(s) on the answer form by filling the circle(s). You have a total of **4 prescriptions** in this station.

This station must be completed in 6 minutes

Written Rx 1

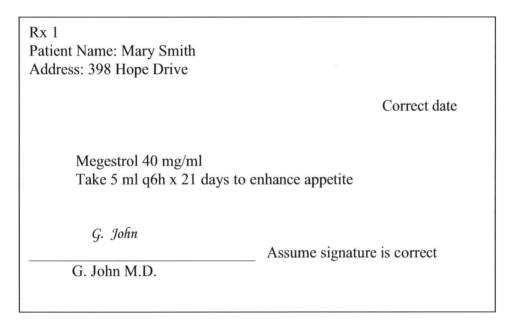

Rx 1
Patient Name: Mary Smith
Address: 398 Hope Drive

Correct date

Megestrol 40 mg/ml
Take 5 ml q6h x 21 days to enhance appetite

G. John
_____   Assume signature is correct
G. John M.D.

Dispensed Rx 1 label

Rx 1   Dr. G. John
Mary Smith
                                        Correct date

Take five milliliters every six hours
for twenty-one days to enhance appetite

Megestrol 40 mg

Rx1: Dispensed Product

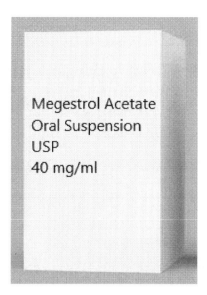

Megestrol Acetate
Oral Suspension
USP
40 mg/ml

Written Rx 2

Rx 2
Patient Name: Jake Min
Address: 340 2nd Street

Correct date

Meloxicam 7.5 mg
2 tabs once a day x 6 weeks

T. Fall

_____ Assume signature is correct
T. Fall M.D.

Dispensed Rx 2 label

Rx 2   Dr. T. Fall
Jaklline Min

                                             Correct date

            Take two tablets once
            a day for five weeks

        Meloxicam 7.5 mg

        84 tablets

Rx2: Dispensed Product

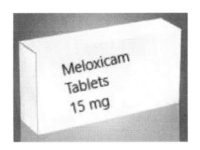

Written Rx 3

Rx 3
Patient Name: Nancy Peter
Address: 2123 Street

                                             Correct date

    Granisetron
    3.1mg patch q5days for 10 days for nausea

        B. Ali
    _____   Assume signature is correct
        B. Ali M.D.

Dispensed Rx 3 label

Rx 3   Dr. B. Ali
Nancy Peter

                                                Correct date

            Take one tablet every five days
            for ten days for nausea

        Granisetron 3.1mg

        2 patches

Rx3: Dispensed Product

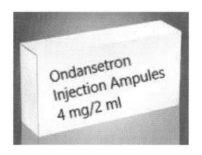

Written Rx 4

Rx 4
Patient Name: Rick Johnson
Address: 2123 Street

                                                Correct date

        Linezolid 100 mg/5ml susp
        300 mg q12h x 14 days for skin infection

        F. Koo
        _____ Assume signature is correct
        F. Koo M.D.

Dispensed Rx 4 label

Rx 4   Dr. F. Koo
Rick Johnson

                                              Correct date

        Take one tablespoon every twelve hours
        for fourteen days for skin infection

        Linezolid 100 mg/ 5ml suspension

Rx4: Dispensed Product

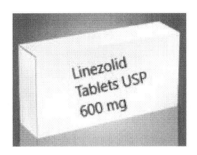

Answer Form #3

Rx1 Dispensed product related problems (refer to enclosed images)	Rx1 Label related problems
O Drug ID O Drug dosage form O Drug strength O Drug packaging O No product problem	O Physician name O Patient name O Drug name O Drug quantity Ø Drug strength O Drug dosage form O Directions of use O No label problem
Rx2 Dispensed product related problems (refer to enclosed images)	Rx2 Label related problems (refer to enclosed Rx label)
O Drug ID O Drug dosage form Ø Drug strength O Drug packaging O No product problem	O Physician name Ø Patient name O Drug name O Drug quantity O Drug strength O Drug dosage form Ø Directions of use O No label problem
Rx3 Dispensed product related problems (refer to enclosed images)	Rx3 Label related problems (refer to enclosed Rx label)
O Drug ID O Drug dosage form O Drug strength O Drug packaging O No product problem	O Physician name O Patient name O Drug name O Drug quantity O Drug strength O Drug dosage form O Directions of use

	O No label problem
Rx4 Dispensed product related problems (refer to enclosed images)	Rx4 Label related problems (refer to enclosed Rx label)
O Drug ID Ø Drug dosage form Ø Drug strength O Drug packaging O No product problem	O Physician name O Patient name O Drug name O Drug quantity O Drug strength O Drug dosage form O Directions of use (before meals – ac) Ø No label problem

Answer Key #3

Rx1 Dispensed product related problems (refer to enclosed images)	**Rx1** Label related problems
○ Drug ID ○ Drug dosage form ○ Drug strength ○ Drug packaging ● **No product problem**	○ Physician name ○ Patient name ○ Drug name ○ Drug quantity ● **Drug strength (40mg/ml)** ○ Drug dosage form ○ Directions of use ○ No label problem
Rx2 Dispensed product related problems (refer to enclosed images)	**Rx2** Label related problems (refer to enclosed Rx label)
○ Drug ID ○ Drug dosage form ● **Drug strength** ○ Drug packaging ○ No product problem	○ Physician name ● **Patient name** ○ Drug name ○ Drug quantity ○ Drug strength ○ Drug dosage form ● **Directions of use (duration of treatment)** ○ No label problem
Rx3 Dispensed product related problems (refer to enclosed images)	**Rx3** Label related problems (refer to enclosed Rx label)
● **Drug ID** ● **Drug dosage form** ○ Drug strength ○ Drug packaging ○ No product problem	○ Physician name ○ Patient name ○ Drug name ○ Drug quantity ○ Drug strength ○ Drug dosage form

	• **Directions of use (administration route)** O No label problem
Rx4 Dispensed product related problems (refer to enclosed images)	**Rx4** Label related problems (refer to enclosed Rx label)
O Drug ID • **Drug dosage form** • **Drug strength** O Drug packaging O No product problem	O Physician name O Patient name O Drug name O Drug quantity O Drug strength O Drug dosage form O Directions of use • **No label problem**

Non-interactive Station #4: Dispensed Prescriptions Check

Candidate's instructions:

Identify any problem(s) related to the dispensed **product** and **label**, **if any**, that must be corrected prior to releasing the product. Mark **all** identified problem(s) on the answer form by filling the circle(s). You have a total of **4 prescriptions** in this station.

This station must be completed in 6 minutes

Written Rx 1

Rx 1
Patient Name: Lory Sunny
Address: 344 Eagle Street

Correct date

Acitretin
25 mg cap po once a day x 7 days

K, John

_____   Assume signature is correct
K. John M.D.

Dispensed Rx 1 label

Rx 1   Dr. K. John
Lory Sunny
Correct date

Take one capsule daily for seven days

Bacitretin 25 mg
7 tablets

Rx1: Dispensed Product

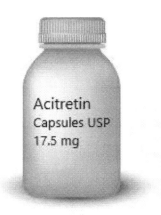

Acitretin
Capsules USP
17.5 mg

Written Rx 2

Rx 2
Patient Name: Pamela Malik
Address: 34A Rain Court

Correct date

Amitriptyline
50 mg once a day for 8 weeks

N. Smith

_____   Assume signature is correct
N. Smith M.D.

Dispensed Rx 2 label

Rx 2   Dr. N. Smith
Pamela Malik

Correct date

Take one tablet once
a day for eight weeks

Amitriptyline 25 mg

102 tablets

Rx2: Dispensed Product

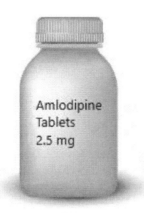

Written Rx 3

```
Rx 3
Patient Name: Frank Paul
Address: 55-2nd Street

                                        Correct date


      Atovaquone 750 mg/ 5ml
      5 ml bid for 21 days


         F. Bryan
   _____   Assume signature is correct
        F. Bryan M.D.
```

Dispensed Rx 3 label

```
Rx 3                              Dr. F. Bryan
Frank Paul
                                 Correct date


          Take one tablespoon twice a day
          for twenty-one days


       Atovaquone 75 mg/ 5ml suspension
```

Rx 3: Dispensed Product

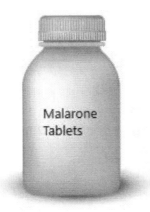

250 mg Atovaquone and 100 mg proguanil HCl Tablets

Written Rx 4

Rx 4
Patient Name: Veronique Smith
Address: 3 Hope Street

                                        Correct date

Glycopyrrolate 0.2 mg/ml
0.1 mg IM qid at 4h intervals for peptic ulcer for one week

K, John
_____ Assume signature is correct
K. John M.D.

Dispensed Rx 4 label

Rx 4   Dr. K. John
Veronique Smith
                                        Correct date

Take one tablet four times a day at 4
hours intervals for peptic ulcer for one
week

Glycopyrrolate 1 mg

28 tablets

Rx4: Dispensed Product

Glycopyrrolate 1 mg tablet

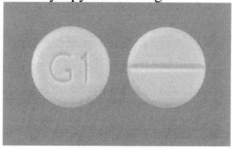

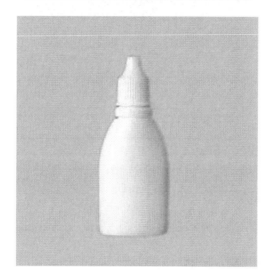

Answer Form #4

Rx1 Dispensed product related problems (refer to enclosed images)	Rx1 Label related problems
O Drug ID O Drug dosage form Ø Drug strength O Drug packaging O No product problem	O Physician name O Patient name ⊙ Drug name O Drug quantity Ø Drug strength O Drug dosage form O Directions of use O No label problem
Rx2 Dispensed product related problems (refer to enclosed images)	Rx2 Label related problems (refer to enclosed Rx label)
O Drug ID O Drug dosage form O Drug strength O Drug packaging O No product problem	O Physician name O Patient name O Drug name O Drug quantity O Drug strength O Drug dosage form O Directions of use O No label problem
Rx3 Dispensed product related problems (refer to enclosed images)	Rx3 Label related problems (refer to enclosed Rx label)
⊙ Drug ID ⊙ Drug dosage form O Drug strength O Drug packaging O No product problem	O Physician name O Patient name O Drug name O Drug quantity ⊙ Drug strength ⊙ Drug dosage form ⊙ Directions of use

	O No label problem
Rx4 Dispensed product related problems (refer to enclosed images)	Rx4 Label related problems (refer to enclosed Rx label)
O Drug ID O Drug dosage form O Drug strength O Drug packaging O No product problem	O Physician name O Patient name O Drug name O Drug quantity O Drug strength O Drug dosage form O Directions of use (before meals – ac) O No label problem

Answer Key #4

Rx1 Dispensed product related problems (refer to enclosed images)	**Rx1** Label related problems
O Drug ID O Drug dosage form ● **Drug strength** O Drug packaging O No product problem	O Physician name O Patient name ● **Drug name** O Drug quantity O Drug strength O Drug dosage form O Directions of use O No label problem
Rx2 Dispensed product related problems (refer to enclosed images)	**Rx2** Label related problems (refer to enclosed Rx label)
● **Drug ID** O Drug dosage form ● **Drug strength** O Drug packaging O No product problem	O Physician name O Patient name O Drug name ● **Drug quantity (112 tablets)** O Drug strength O Drug dosage form ● **Directions of use (take 2 tablets)** O No label problem
Rx3 Dispensed product related problems (refer to enclosed images)	**Rx3** Label related problems (refer to enclosed Rx label)
● **Drug ID (malarone is a combination of atovaquone and proguanil)** ● **Drug dosage form** O Drug strength O Drug packaging O No product problem	O Physician name O Patient name O Drug name O Drug quantity ● **Drug strength** O Drug dosage form ● **Directions of use (take 1 teaspoon)** O No label problem

Rx4 Dispensed product related problems (refer to enclosed images)	**Rx4** Label related problems (refer to enclosed Rx label)
O Drug ID ● **Drug dosage form** O Drug strength ● **Drug packaging** O No product problem	O Physician name O Patient name O Drug name O Drug quantity O Drug strength ● **Drug dosage form** O Directions of use O No label problem

Non-interactive Station #5: Dispensed Prescriptions Check

Candidate's instructions:

Identify any problem(s) related to the dispensed **product** and **label**, **if any**, that must be corrected prior to releasing the product. Mark **all** identified problem(s) on the answer form by filling the circle(s). You have a total of **4 prescriptions** in this station.

This station must be completed in 6 minutes

Written Rx 1

Rx 1
Patient Name: Marie Simon
Address: 3 Marmot Road

Correct date

Atorvastatin
Start at 10mg daily, increase by 10 mg every 2 weeks up to 50 mg daily then continue at 50 mg daily for 4 weeks

P. Wang

_____ Assume signature is correct
P. Wang M.D.

Dispensed Rx 1 label

Rx 1   Dr. K. Wang
Marie Simon
                                      Correct date

Take one tablet daily for two weeks
Then two tablets for two more weeks
Then 3 tablets for two more weeks
Then 4 tablets for two more weeks
Then 5 tablets for four more weeks

Atorvastatin 10 mg

282 tablets

Rx1: Dispensed Product

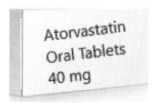

Written Rx 2

Rx 2
Patient Name: Renee Wayne
Address: 34 Major Road

                                              Correct date

Nevirapine
200 mg once a day x 14 days
then increase to 200 mg bid x 4 weeks

W. Arthur
_____ Assume signature is correct
        W. Arthur M.D.

Dispensed Rx 2 label

Rx 2   Dr. N. Smith
Renee White
                                        Correct date

    Take two tablets once a day for 14 days
    Then take one tablet twice a day for four weeks

    Nebirapine 200mg

    70 tablets

Rx2: Dispensed Product

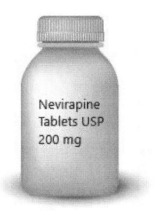

Nevirapine
Tablets USP
200 mg

Written Rx 3

Rx 3
Patient Name: Fanny Koo
Address: 2123 Street

Correct date

Nifedipine
20 mg cap tid x 3 weeks for angina

F. Thomas

_____ Assume signature is correct
F. Thomas M.D.

Dispensed Rx 3 label

Rx 3   Dr. F. Thomas
Fanny Koo
                                             Correct date

Take one capsule three times a day
for three weeks for angina

Nifedipine 20 mg

63 tablets

Rx3: Dispensed Product

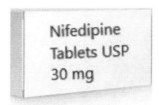

Written Rx 4

Rx 4
Patient Name: Tannis John
Address: 34A Street

Correct date

Prednisolone
5 mg tab bid cc x 30 days

Y. Smith
_____   Assume signature is correct
Y. Smith M.D.

Dispensed Rx 4 label

Rx 4   Dr. Y. Smith
Tannis John
                                      Correct date

Take one tablet twice a day for 30 days

Prednisolone 5 mg

60 tablets

Rx4: Dispensed Product

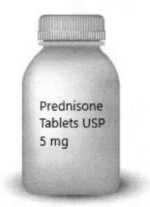

Prednisone
Tablets USP
5 mg

Answer Form #5

Rx1 Dispensed product related problems (refer to enclosed images)	Rx1 Label related problems
O Drug ID O Drug dosage form ⊘ Drug strength O Drug packaging O No product problem	⊘ Physician name O Patient name O Drug name O Drug quantity O Drug strength O Drug dosage form O Directions of use O No label problem
Rx2 Dispensed product related problems (refer to enclosed images)	**Rx2 Label related problems (refer to enclosed Rx label)**
⊘ Drug ID O Drug dosage form O Drug strength O Drug packaging ⊘ No product problem	O Physician name ⊘ Patient name ⊘ Drug name O Drug quantity O Drug strength O Drug dosage form ⊘ Directions of use O No label problem
Rx3 Dispensed product related problems (refer to enclosed images)	**Rx3 Label related problems (refer to enclosed Rx label)**
O Drug ID ⊘ Drug dosage form Capsules not tab ⊘ Drug strength O Drug packaging O No product problem	O Physician name O Patient name O Drug name O Drug quantity O Drug strength O Drug dosage form O Directions of use

Rx4 Dispensed product related problems (refer to enclosed images)	Rx4 Label related problems (refer to enclosed Rx label)
	O No label problem
☑ Drug ID O Drug dosage form O Drug strength O Drug packaging O No product problem	O Physician name O Patient name O Drug name O Drug quantity O Drug strength O Drug dosage form ☑ Directions of use (before meals – ac) O No label problem

Answer Key #5

Rx1 Dispensed product related problems (refer to enclosed images)	**Rx1** Label related problems
○ Drug ID ○ Drug dosage form ● **Drug strength** ○ Drug packaging ○ No product problem	● **Physician name** ○ Patient name ○ Drug name ● **Drug quantity (280 tablets)** ○ Drug strength ○ Drug dosage form ○ Directions of use ○ No label problem
Rx2 Dispensed product related problems (refer to enclosed images)	**Rx2** Label related problems (refer to enclosed Rx label)
○ Drug ID ○ Drug dosage form ○ Drug strength ○ Drug packaging ● **No product problem**	○ Physician name ○ Patient name ● **Drug name** ○ Drug quantity ○ Drug strength ○ Drug dosage form ● **Directions of use (take one tablet for 14 days)** ○ No label problem
Rx3 Dispensed product related problems (refer to enclosed images)	**Rx3** Label related problems (refer to enclosed Rx label)
○ Drug ID ● **Drug dosage form** ● **Drug strength** ○ Drug packaging ○ No product problem	○ Physician name ○ Patient name ○ Drug name ○ Drug quantity ○ Drug strength ○ Drug dosage form ○ Directions of use

	● **No label problem**
Rx4 Dispensed product related problems (refer to enclosed images)	**Rx4** Label related problems (refer to enclosed Rx label)
● **Drug ID** O Drug dosage form O Drug strength O Drug packaging O No product problem	O Physician name O Patient name O Drug name O Drug quantity O Drug strength O Drug dosage form ● **Directions of use (add with meals-cc)** O No label problem

Non-interactive Case #6: Dispensed Prescriptions Check

Candidate's instructions:

Identify any problem(s) related to the dispensed **product** and **label**, **if any**, that must be corrected prior to releasing the product. Mark **all** identified problem(s) on the answer form by filling the circle(s). You have a total of **4 prescriptions** in this station.

This station must be completed in 6 minutes

Written Rx 1

Rx 1
Patient Name: Art Smith
Address: 300 Hope Road

Correct date

Atorvastatin
40 mg daily x 6weeks

K. John
_____   Assume signature is correct
K. John M.D.

Dispensed Rx 1 label

Rx 1   Dr. K. John
Art Smith
                                        Correct date

Take one tablet once a day
for six weeks

Atorvastatin 40 mg
42 tablets

Rx1: Dispensed Product

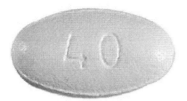

Atorvastatin 40 mg

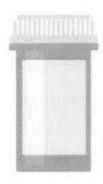

Written Rx 2

Rx 2
Patient Name: Linda Shims
Address: 355A Street

Correct date

Oxacillin 250 mg/5 ml
500 mg q4h x 10 days

N. Joy

_____   Assume signature is correct
N. Joy M.D.

Dispensed Rx 2 label

Rx 2   Dr. N. Joy
Linda Shims
                                         Correct date

Take two tablespoons every four hours
for ten days

Oxacillin 250 mg/ ml

Rx2: Dispensed Product

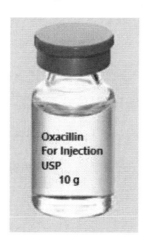

Oxacillin
For Injection
USP
10 g

Written Rx 3

Rx 3
Patient Name: Tim Low
Address: 21B Street

                                                                 Correct date

      Mesalamine 500 mg
      1 supp pr bid x 6 weeks for ulcerative colitis

       F. Kassam
_____ Assume signature is correct
      F. Kassam M.D.

Dispensed Rx 3 label

Rx 3   Dr. F. Kassam
Tim Low

                             Correct date

          Take one tablet twice a day
          for six weeks

      Mesamine 500 mg

      84 tablets

Rx3: Dispensed Product

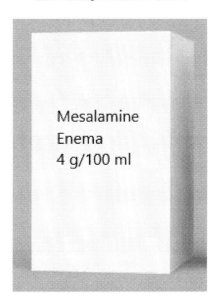

Mesalamine
Enema
4 g/100 ml

Written Rx 4

Rx 4
Patient Name: Jamie Scott
Address: 212 Vancouver Street

Correct date

Methylphenidate SR
20 mg once a day before breakfast for 2 wks for ADD

P. Thomas

_____ Assume signature is correct
P. Thomas M.D.

Dispensed Rx 4 label

Rx 4   Dr. P. Thomas
Jamie Scott

                                        Correct date

   Take one tablet once a day before breakfast
   for two weeks for Attention Deficit Disorder

   Methylphenidate 20 mg

      14 tablets

Rx4: Dispensed Product

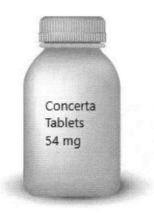

Concerta
Tablets
54 mg

Answer Form #6

Rx1 Dispensed product related problems (refer to enclosed images)	Rx1 Label related problems
O Drug ID O Drug dosage form O Drug strength O Drug packaging Ⓞ No product problem	O Physician name O Patient name O Drug name O Drug quantity O Drug strength O Drug dosage form O Directions of use Ⓞ No label problem
Rx2 Dispensed product related problems (refer to enclosed images)	Rx2 Label related problems (refer to enclosed Rx label)
O Drug ID Ⓞ Drug dosage form O Drug strength O Drug packaging O No product problem	O Physician name O Patient name O Drug name O Drug quantity Ⓞ Drug strength O Drug dosage form Ⓞ Directions of use O No label problem
Rx3 Dispensed product related problems (refer to enclosed images)	Rx3 Label related problems (refer to enclosed Rx label)
O Drug ID Ⓞ Drug dosage form Ⓞ Drug strength O Drug packaging O No product problem	O Physician name O Patient name Ⓞ Drug name O Drug quantity O Drug strength Ⓞ Drug dosage form O Directions of use

123

	O No label problem
Rx4 Dispensed product related problems (refer to enclosed images)	Rx4 Label related problems (refer to enclosed Rx label)
O Drug ID O Drug dosage form O Drug strength O Drug packaging O No product problem	O Physician name O Patient name O Drug name O Drug quantity O Drug strength O Drug dosage form O Directions of use (before meals – ac) O No label problem

Answer Key #6

Rx1 Dispensed product related problems (refer to enclosed images)	**Rx1** Label related problems
O Drug ID O Drug dosage form O Drug strength O Drug packaging ● **No product problem**	O Physician name O Patient name O Drug name O Drug quantity O Drug strength O Drug dosage form O Directions of use ● **No label problem**
Rx2 Dispensed product related problems (refer to enclosed images)	**Rx2** Label related problems (refer to enclosed Rx label)
O Drug ID ● **Drug dosage form** O Drug strength O Drug packaging O No product problem	O Physician name O Patient name O Drug name O Drug quantity ● **Drug strength (250 mg/5ml)** O Drug dosage form ● **Directions of use (take 2 teaspoons)** O No label problem
Rx3 Dispensed product related problems (refer to enclosed images)	**Rx3** Label related problems (refer to enclosed Rx label)
O Drug ID ● **Drug dosage form** O Drug strength O Drug packaging O No product problem	O Physician name O Patient name ● **Drug name** O Drug quantity O Drug strength ● **Drug dosage form**

	• **Directions of use (administration route)** O No label problem
Rx4 Dispensed product related problems (refer to enclosed images)	**Rx4** Label related problems (refer to enclosed Rx label)
O Drug ID O Drug dosage form • **Drug strength** O Drug packaging O No product problem	O Physician name O Patient name O Drug name O Drug quantity O Drug strength • **Drug dosage form (add SR)** O Directions of use O No label problem

126

Non-interactive Station #7: Dispensed Prescriptions Check

Candidate's instructions:

Identify any problem(s) related to the dispensed **product** and **label**, **if any**, that must be corrected prior to releasing the product. Mark **all** identified problem(s) on the answer form by filling the circle(s). You have a total of **4 prescriptions** in this station.

This station must be completed in 6 minutes

Written Rx 1

Rx 1
Patient Name: Veronica Smith
Address: 3 Hope Street

Correct date

Meloxicam
15 mg once a day x 8 weeks for RA

T. Young
_____ Assume signature is correct
T. Young M.D.

Dispensed Rx 1 label

Rx 1   Dr. T. Young
Veronica Smith
                                        Correct date

        Take one tablet once a day for eight
        weeks for rheumatoid arthritis

    Meloxicam 7.5 mg

    56 tablets

Rx1: Dispensed Product

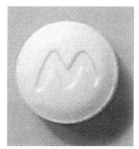

Meloxicam 15 mg

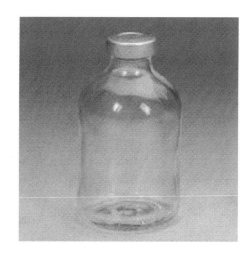

Written Rx 2

Rx 2
Patient Name: Pamela Moon
Address: 388A Sunny Road

Correct date

Mefloquine
250 mg once/wk x 4 wks
Then 250 mg every other wk x 10 wks

N. Smith

_____ Assume signature is correct
N. Smith M.D.

Dispensed Rx 2 label

Rx 2   Dr. N. Smith
Pamela Moon
                                        Correct date

Take one tablet once each week for four
weeks then one tablet every other week
for ten weeks

Melfaquine 250 mg

9 tablets

Rx2: Dispensed Product

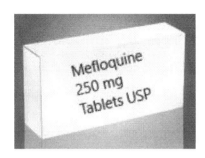

Written Rx 3

Rx 3
Patient Name: Jimmy Pete
Address: 21st Street

Correct date

Flavoxate
100 mg po tid x 30 days for incontinence

F. Smith
_____   Assume signature is correct
F. Smith M.D.

Dispensed Rx 3 label

Rx 3   Dr. F. Smith
Janny Pete

Correct date

Take one tablet three times a day
for 30 days for incontinence

Flavoxate 100 g

90 tablets

<u>Rx3: Dispensed Product</u>

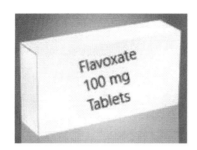

Written Rx 4

Rx 4
Patient Name: Halim Parker
Address: 34C Seaview Court

                                            Correct date

Sulfamethoxazole/Trimethoprim 200 mg SMX/40 mg TMP/ 5ml
Equivalent child dose of adult 800 mg SMX/160 mg TMP q12h x
7 days for infection assuming a child BSA of 0.75 m^2

N. Smith
_____   Assume signature is correct
      N. Smith M.D.

Dispensed Rx 4 label

Rx 4   Dr. N. Sam
Halim Parker
                                        Correct date

                  Take 7.5 ml every twelve hours
                   for seven days for infection

                 Sulfamethoxazole/Trimethoprim
              200 mg SMX/40 mg TMP/ 5ml suspension

Rx4: Dispensed Product

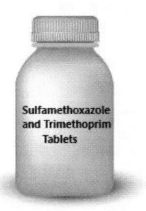

Sulfamethoxazole and Trimethoprim Tablets

Answer Form #7

Rx1 Dispensed product related problems (refer to enclosed images)	Rx1 Label related problems
O Drug ID O Drug dosage form O Drug strength O Drug packaging O No product problem	O Physician name O Patient name O Drug name O Drug quantity O Drug strength O Drug dosage form O Directions of use O No label problem
Rx2 Dispensed product related problems (refer to enclosed images)	Rx2 Label related problems (refer to enclosed Rx label)
O Drug ID O Drug dosage form O Drug strength O Drug packaging O No product problem	O Physician name O Patient name O Drug name O Drug quantity O Drug strength O Drug dosage form O Directions of use O No label problem
Rx3 Dispensed product related problems (refer to enclosed images)	Rx3 Label related problems (refer to enclosed Rx label)
O Drug ID O Drug dosage form O Drug strength O Drug packaging O No product problem	O Physician name O Patient name O Drug name O Drug quantity O Drug strength O Drug dosage form O Directions of use

	O No label problem
Rx4 Dispensed product related problems (refer to enclosed images)	Rx4 Label related problems (refer to enclosed Rx label)
O Drug ID O Drug dosage form O Drug strength O Drug packaging O No product problem	O Physician name O Patient name O Drug name O Drug quantity O Drug strength O Drug dosage form O Directions of use (before meals – ac) O No label problem

Answer Key #7

Rx1 Dispensed product related problems (refer to enclosed images)	**Rx1** Label related problems
O Drug ID O Drug dosage form O Drug strength ● **Drug packaging** O No product problem	O Physician name O Patient name O Drug name O Drug quantity ● **Drug strength** O Drug dosage form O Directions of use O No label problem
Rx2 Dispensed product related problems (refer to enclosed images)	**Rx2** Label related problems (refer to enclosed Rx label)
O Drug ID O Drug dosage form O Drug strength O Drug packaging ● **No product problem**	O Physician name O Patient name ● **Drug name** O Drug quantity O Drug strength O Drug dosage form O Directions of use O No label problem
Rx3 Dispensed product related problems (refer to enclosed images)	**Rx3** Label related problems (refer to enclosed Rx label)
O Drug ID O Drug dosage form O Drug strength O Drug packaging ● **No product problem**	O Physician name ● **Patient name** O Drug name O Drug quantity ● **Drug strength (100 mg)** O Drug dosage form O Directions of use

	○ No label problem
Rx4 Dispensed product related problems (refer to enclosed images)	**Rx4** Label related problems (refer to enclosed Rx label)

○ Drug ID
 	
  ● **Drug dosage form**
 	
  ○ Drug strength
 	
  ○ Drug packaging
 	
  ○ No product problem
	● **Physician name**
	
	  ○ Patient name
	
	  ○ Drug name
	
	  ○ Drug quantity
	
	  ○ Drug strength
	
	  ○ Drug dosage form
	
	  ● **Directions of use**
	Dose (child) = [BSA (child) / BSA (adult)] x Dose (adult)
	BSA (adult) = 1.73 m^2
	Correct dose is 8.6 ml
	
	  ○ No label problem

Non-interactive Station #8: Dispensed Prescriptions Check

Candidate's instructions:

Identify any problem(s) related to the dispensed **product** and **label**, **if any**, that must be corrected prior to releasing the product. Mark **all** identified problem(s) on the answer form by filling the circle(s). You have a total of **4 prescriptions** in this station.

<u>This station must be completed in 6 minutes</u>

Written Rx 1

Rx 1
Patient Name: Veronique George
Address: 311 Hope Street

Correct date

Timolol 0.25% sol
1 drp od bid x 7 days

K. Lee

_____   Assume signature is correct
K. Lee M.D.

Dispensed Rx 1 label

Rx 1   Dr. K. Lee
Veronique George
                                          Correct date

Place one drop in each eye
twice a day for seven days

Timolol 0.25% gel

Rx1: Dispensed Product

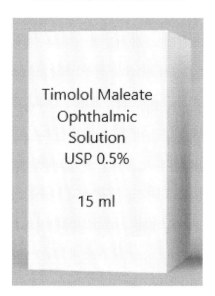

Timolol Maleate
Ophthalmic
Solution
USP 0.5%

15 ml

Written Rx 2

Rx 2
Patient Name: Marie Henry
Address: 3 Montreal Street

Correct date

Lamotrigine
50 mg once a day x 2 wks
Then 50 mg bid x 2 wks
Then increase by 100 mg daily at 2 wks interval until 300 mg bid
Then continue at 300 mg bid for 5 wks

A. Peter

_____ Assume signature is correct
A. Peter M.D.

Dispensed Rx 2 label

Rx 2   Dr. A. Peter

Marie Henry

                                       Correct date

Take one tablet once a day for fourteen days
Then take one tablet twice a day for fourteen days
Then take two tablets twice a day for fourteen days
Then take three tablets twice a day for thirty-five days

Lamotrigine 50 mg

308 tablets

Rx2: Dispensed Product

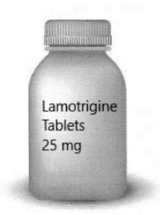

Written Rx 3

Rx 3
Patient Name: Fiona Dakota
Address: 2123 3rd Road

Correct date

Methimazole
5 mg tab q8h x 6 weeks for hyperthyroidism

F. Hakim
_____   Assume signature is correct
F. Hakim M.D.

Dispensed Rx 3 label

Rx 3   Dr. F. Hakim
Fiona Dakota

Correct date

Take one tablet every eight hours
for six weeks for hyperthyroidism

Methimazole 5 mg

128 tablets

Rx3: Dispensed Product

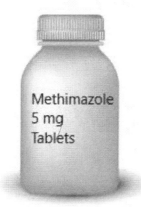

139

Written Rx 4

Rx 4
Patient Name: Rene Paul
Address: 35 Fox Street

Correct date

Tetracycline 125 mg/5ml susp
250 mg tid x 10 days

L. Liam
_____   Assume signature is correct
L. Liam M.D.

Dispensed Rx 4 label

Rx 4   Dr. L. Liam
Rene Paul ✓

Correct date

Take two teaspoons three times a day for ten
days

Tetracycline 125mg/ml suspension

Rx4: Dispensed Product

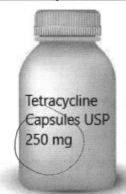

Tetracycline
Capsules USP
250 mg

Answer Form #8

Rx1 Dispensed product related problems (refer to enclosed images)	Rx1 Label related problems
O Drug ID O Drug dosage form O Drug strength O Drug packaging O No product problem	O Physician name O Patient name O Drug name O Drug quantity O Drug strength O Drug dosage form O Directions of use O No label problem
Rx2 Dispensed product related problems (refer to enclosed images)	Rx2 Label related problems (refer to enclosed Rx label)
O Drug ID O Drug dosage form O Drug strength O Drug packaging O No product problem	O Physician name O Patient name O Drug name O Drug quantity O Drug strength O Drug dosage form O Directions of use O No label problem
Rx3 Dispensed product related problems (refer to enclosed images)	Rx3 Label related problems (refer to enclosed Rx label)
O Drug ID O Drug dosage form O Drug strength O Drug packaging O No product problem	O Physician name O Patient name O Drug name O Drug quantity O Drug strength O Drug dosage form O Directions of use

	O No label problem
Rx4 Dispensed product related problems (refer to enclosed images)	Rx4 Label related problems (refer to enclosed Rx label)
O Drug ID O Drug dosage form O Drug strength O Drug packaging O No product problem	O Physician name O Patient name O Drug name O Drug quantity O Drug strength O Drug dosage form O Directions of use (before meals – ac) O No label problem

Answer Key #8

Rx1 Dispensed product related problems (refer to enclosed images)	**Rx1** Label related problems
O Drug ID O Drug dosage form ● **Drug strength** O Drug packaging O No product problem	O Physician name O Patient name O Drug name O Drug quantity O Drug strength ● **Drug dosage form** ● **Directions of use (right eye)** O No label problem
Rx2 Dispensed product related problems (refer to enclosed images)	**Rx2** Label related problems (refer to enclosed Rx label)
O Drug ID O Drug dosage form ● **Drug strength** O Drug packaging O No product problem	O Physician name O Patient name O Drug name O Drug quantity O Drug strength O Drug dosage form O Directions of use ● **No label problem**
Rx3 Dispensed product related problems (refer to enclosed images)	**Rx3** Label related problems (refer to enclosed Rx label)
O Drug ID O Drug dosage form O Drug strength O Drug packaging ● **No product problem**	O Physician name O Patient name O Drug name ● **Drug quantity (126 tablets)** O Drug strength O Drug dosage form O Directions of use O No label problem

Rx4 Dispensed product related problems (refer to enclosed images)	**Rx4** Label related problems (refer to enclosed Rx label)
O Drug ID	O Physician name
● **Drug dosage form**	O Patient name
O Drug strength	O Drug name
O Drug packaging	O Drug quantity
O No product problem	● **Drug strength (125 mg/5 ml)**
	O Drug dosage form
	O Directions of use
	O No label problem

Non-interactive case #9: Dispensed Prescriptions Check

Candidate's instructions:

Identify any problem(s) related to the dispensed **product** and **label**, **if any**, that must be corrected prior to releasing the product. Mark **all** identified problem(s) on the answer form by filling the circle(s). You have a total of **4 prescriptions** in this station.

This station must be completed in 6 minutes

Written Rx 1

Rx 1
Patient Name: Rory May
Address: 21 Calgary Avenue

Correct date

Sulfadiazine 500 mg tabs
150 mg/kg/day divided in 4 doses (4g/day max) for 5 days
Child weight is 30 kg

F. Wang

_____   Assume signature is correct
F. Wang M.D.

Dispensed Rx 1 label

Rx 1   Dr. F.Wang
Rory May
                                        Correct date

Take two tablets four times a day
for five days

Sulfadiazine 500 mg

40 tablets

Rx1: Dispensed Product

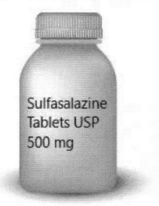

Sulfasalazine
Tablets USP
500 mg

Written Rx 2

Rx 2
Patient Name: Roger Smith
Address: 35 Hill Street

Correct date

Meperidine HCl 50 mg/5ml syrup
1.5 mg/kg q4h (max: 100 mg q4h) prn for pain
Child weight is 50 kg

K. Junior

_____   Assume signature is correct
     K. Junior M.D.

Dispensed Rx 2 label

Rx 2   Dr. K. Junior
Roger Smith

Correct date

Take one tablespoon every four hours as
needed for pain

Meperidine HCl 50 mg/5ml syrup

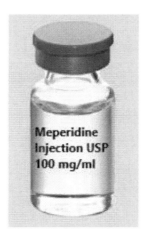

Written Rx 3

Rx 3
Patient Name: Cathy Fong
Address: 21 2nd street

                                                                    Correct date

    Efavirenz
    600 mg tablet daily x 90 days

      H. Kong
_____   Assume signature is correct
    H. Kong M.D.

Dispensed Rx 3 label

Rx 3   Dr. H. Kong
Cathy Fong
                                                        Correct date

        Take one tablet daily for 90 days

     Efavirenz 600 mg

    90 tablets

Rx3: Dispensed Product

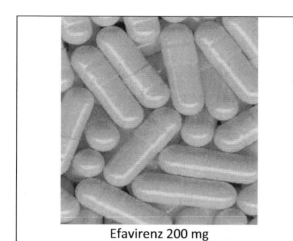

Efavirenz 200 mg

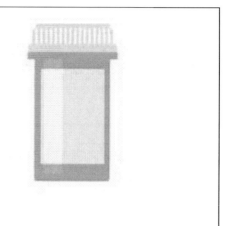

Written Rx 4

Rx 4
Patient Name: Kim Don
Address: 21 Green Street

Correct date

Captopril
50 mg tid x 2 weeks

A. Hammond

_____   Assume signature is correct
A. Hammond M.D.

Dispensed Rx 4 label

Rx 4   Dr. A. Hammond
Kim Don

Correct date

Take two tablets three times
a day for two weeks

Captopril 25 mg

78 tablets

Rx4: Dispensed Product

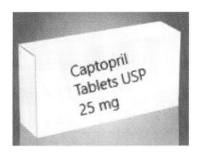

Answer Form #9

Rx1 Dispensed product related problems (refer to enclosed images)	Rx1 Label related problems
O Drug ID O Drug dosage form O Drug strength O Drug packaging O No product problem	O Physician name O Patient name O Drug name O Drug quantity O Drug strength O Drug dosage form O Directions of use O No label problem
Rx2 Dispensed product related problems (refer to enclosed images)	Rx2 Label related problems (refer to enclosed Rx label)
O Drug ID O Drug dosage form O Drug strength O Drug packaging O No product problem	O Physician name O Patient name O Drug name O Drug quantity O Drug strength O Drug dosage form O Directions of use O No label problem
Rx3 Dispensed product related problems (refer to enclosed images)	Rx3 Label related problems (refer to enclosed Rx label)
O Drug ID O Drug dosage form O Drug strength O Drug packaging O No product problem	O Physician name O Patient name O Drug name O Drug quantity O Drug strength O Drug dosage form

	O Directions of use
	O No label problem
Rx4 Dispensed product related problems (refer to enclosed images)	Rx4 Label related problems (refer to enclosed Rx label)
O Drug ID	O Physician name
O Drug dosage form	O Patient name
O Drug strength	O Drug name
O Drug packaging	O Drug quantity
O No product problem	O Drug strength
	O Drug dosage form
	O Directions of use (before meals – ac)
	O No label problem

Answer Key #9

Rx1 Dispensed product related problems (refer to enclosed images)	**Rx1** Label related problems
● **Drug ID** ○ Drug dosage form ○ Drug strength ○ Drug packaging ○ No product problem	○ Physician name ○ Patient name ○ Drug name ○ Drug quantity ○ Drug strength ○ Drug dosage form ○ Directions of use ● **No label problem**
Rx2 Dispensed product related problems (refer to enclosed images)	**Rx2** Label related problems (refer to enclosed Rx label)
○ Drug ID ● **Drug dosage form** ● **Drug strength** ○ Drug packaging ○ No product problem	○ Physician name ○ Patient name ○ Drug name ○ Drug quantity ○ Drug strength ○ Drug dosage form ● **Directions of use (take ½ tbsp = 7.5 ml)** ○ No label problem
Rx3 Dispensed product related problems (refer to enclosed images)	**Rx3** Label related problems (refer to enclosed Rx label)
○ Drug ID ● **Drug dosage form (tablets not capsules)** ● **Drug strength** ○ Drug packaging ○ No product problem	○ Physician name ○ Patient name ○ Drug name ○ Drug quantity ○ Drug strength ○ Drug dosage form ○ Directions of use

	● **No label problem**
Rx4 Dispensed product related problems (refer to enclosed images)	**Rx4** Label related problems (refer to enclosed Rx label)
O Drug ID O Drug dosage form O Drug strength O Drug packaging (if applicable) ● **No product problem**	O Physician name O Patient name O Drug name ● **Drug quantity (84 tablets)** O Drug strength O Drug dosage form O Directions of use O No label problem

Non-interactive case #10: Dispensed Prescriptions Check

Candidate's instructions:

Identify any problem(s) related to the dispensed **product** and **label**, **if any**, that must be corrected prior to releasing the product. Mark **all** identified problem(s) on the answer form by filling the circle(s). You have a total of **4 prescriptions** in this station.

This station must be completed in 6 minutes

Written Rx 1

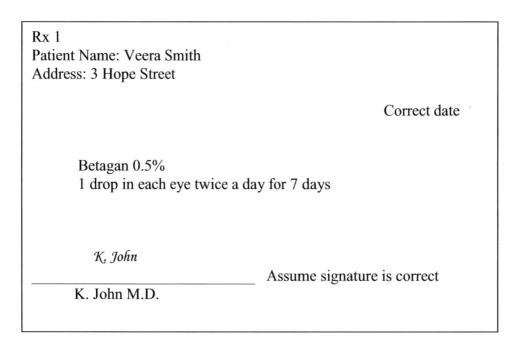

Rx 1
Patient Name: Veera Smith
Address: 3 Hope Street

Correct date

Betagan 0.5%
1 drop in each eye twice a day for 7 days

K. John
_____   Assume signature is correct
K. John M.D.

Dispensed Rx 1 label

Rx 1   Dr. K. John
Veera Smith
                                        Correct date

        Place one drop in each eye
        twice a day for seven days

    Betagan 1% solution

Rx1: Dispensed Product

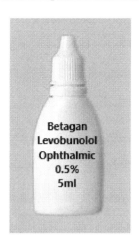

Betagan
Levobunolol
Ophthalmic
0.5%
5ml

Written Rx 2

Rx 2
Patient Name: Tannis Moon
Address: 34A Street

Correct date

Amaryl 1 mg tab
Start with 1 tab once a day, then increase by 1 mg every other
week until 4 mg once daily, then continue for 4 weeks

N. Smith
_____ Assume signature is correct
N. Smith M.D.

Dispensed Rx 2 label

Rx 2   Dr. N. Smith
Tannis Moon
                                        Correct date

Take one tablet once a day for two weeks
Then take two tablets for two more weeks
Then take three tablets for two more weeks
Then take four tablets for four more weeks

Amiryl 1 mg

195 tablets

Rx2: Dispensed Product

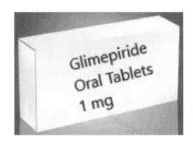

Written Rx 3

Rx 3
Patient Name: Fanny Pete
Address: 2123 Street

                                        Correct date

Zofran 2mg/ml
IV 0.15 mg/kg infused over 15 min beginning
30 min prior to chemotherapy for a 66 lbs child

F. Tom
_____ Assume signature is correct
F. Tom M.D.

Dispensed Rx 3 label

Rx 3   Dr. F. Tom
Fanny Pete
                                        Correct date

        2.25 ml by intravenous infusion over
        fifteen minutes beginning thirty minutes
        before chemotherapy for a sixty-six pounds
        child.

    Zofran 2mg/ml

        2.25 ml

Rx3: Dispensed Product

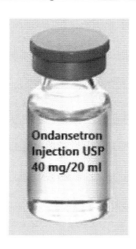

Written Rx 4

Rx 4
Patient Name: Karyn Cains
Address: Moose Street

                                                    Correct date

        Warfarin
        10 mg daily
        Mitte: 30 tablets

            L. Singh
    _____ Assume signature is correct
            L. Singh M.D.

Dispensed Rx 4 label

Rx 4   Dr. L. Singh
Kareen Cains

                                                    Correct date

    Take one tablet daily for thirty days

    Warfarin 10 mg

    30 tablets

Rx4: Dispensed Product

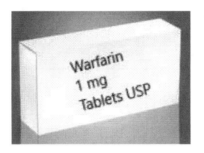

Answer Form #10

Rx1 Dispensed product related problems (refer to enclosed images)	Rx1 Label related problems
O Drug ID O Drug dosage form O Drug strength O Drug packaging O No product problem	O Physician name O Patient name O Drug name O Drug quantity O Drug strength O Drug dosage form O Directions of use O No label problem
Rx2 Dispensed product related problems (refer to enclosed images)	Rx2 Label related problems (refer to enclosed Rx label)
O Drug ID O Drug dosage form O Drug strength O Drug packaging O No product problem	O Physician name O Patient name O Drug name O Drug quantity O Drug strength O Drug dosage form O Directions of use O No label problem
Rx3 Dispensed product related problems (refer to enclosed images)	Rx3 Label related problems (refer to enclosed Rx label)
O Drug ID O Drug dosage form O Drug strength O Drug packaging O No product problem	O Physician name O Patient name O Drug name O Drug quantity O Drug strength O Drug dosage form O Directions of use

	O No label problem
Rx4 Dispensed product related problems (refer to enclosed images)	Rx4 Label related problems (refer to enclosed Rx label)
O Drug ID O Drug dosage form O Drug strength O Drug packaging O No product problem	O Physician name O Patient name O Drug name O Drug quantity O Drug strength O Drug dosage form O Directions of use (before meals – ac) O No label problem

Answer Key #10

Rx1 Dispensed product related problems (refer to enclosed images)	**Rx1** Label related problems
O Drug ID O Drug dosage form O Drug strength O Drug packaging ● **No product problem**	O Physician name O Patient name O Drug name O Drug quantity ● **Drug strength** O Drug dosage form O Directions of use O No label problem
Rx2 Dispensed product related problems (refer to enclosed images)	**Rx2** Label related problems (refer to enclosed Rx label)
O Drug ID O Drug dosage form O Drug strength O Drug packaging ● **No product problem**	O Physician name O Patient name ● **Drug name** ● **Drug quantity (196 tablets)** O Drug strength O Drug dosage form O Directions of use O No label problem
Rx3 Dispensed product related problems (refer to enclosed images)	**Rx3** Label related problems (refer to enclosed Rx label)
O Drug ID O Drug dosage form O Drug strength O Drug packaging ● **No product problem (40 mg/20 ml = 2mg/ml)**	O Physician name O Patient name O Drug name O Drug quantity O Drug strength O Drug dosage form O Directions of use

	● **No label problem**
Rx4 Dispensed product related problems (refer to enclosed images)	**Rx4** Label related problems (refer to enclosed Rx label)
O Drug ID O Drug dosage form ● **Drug strength** O Drug packaging O No product problem	O Physician name ● **Patient name** O Drug name O Drug quantity O Drug strength O Drug dosage form O Directions of use O No label problem

OSPE Non-Interactive Stations

Non-interactive Station #1: Prescriptions/MAR/Blister-Pack Check

Candidate's instructions:

Check the accuracy of the Medication Administration Record (MAR) and Blister-Pack (see below) against the written prescriptions. Record **all** identified mistake(s) and omission(s) on the MAR and Blister-Pack answer form by filling the corresponding circle(s). You have a total of **4 prescriptions** in this station. Note: Make sure to check the shape and shade of tablets, and shade of capsules.

This station must be completed in 6 minutes

Written Prescriptions

Patient Name: Simon Brett
Address: 23th Street, City

Correct date

Rx 1(Drug 1): Lomotil 2.5 mg
    Sig: 2 tablets BID

Rx2 (Drug 2): Sutent 50 mg
    Sig: 1 capsule qd

Rx3 (Drug 3): Synthroid 100 mcg
    Sig: 1 tablet qd

Rx4 (Drug 4): Valcyte 450 mg
    Sig: 2 tablets BID

T. Jeremy
_____ Assume signature is correct
    T. Jeremy M.D.

Medication Administration Record (MAR)

Patient   Simon Brett   **Date of birth**   February 3, 1958
Address   23th Street, City   **Gender**   Male
Phone   555-5555   **Allergies**   None

Physician   Dr. T. Jeremy
Address   4 Wellness Road, City
Phone   888-888

Medications	Description and dosage form	Directions of use	6 AM	NOON	6 PM	HS
Drug 1	Tablet, round white	2 tablets TID	2	2	2	
Drug 2	Capsule	1 capsule BID	1		1	
Drug 3	Tablet, round black	1 tablet qd	1			
Drug 4	Tablet, elongated	2 tablet BID	2			2

164

Blister-Pack

Lomotil ○   Sutent ◖▭◗   Synthroid ●   Xeloda ▭

	AM	NOON	PM	HS
Monday	○ ● ◖▭◗ / ○ ◖▭◗	○ / ○	○ ◖▭◗ / ○	▭ / ▭
Tuesday	○ ● ◖▭◗ / ○ ◖▭◗	○ / ○	○ ◖▭◗ / ○	▭ / ▭
Wednesday	○ ● ◖▭◗ / ○ ◖▭◗	○ / ○	○ ◖▭◗ / ○	▭ / ▭
Thursday	○ ● ◖▭◗ / ○ ◖▭◗	○ / ○	○ ◖▭◗ / ○	▭ / ▭
Friday	○ ● ◖▭◗ / ○ ◖▭◗	○ / ○	○ ◖▭◗ / ○	▭ / ▭
Saturday	○ ● ◖▭◗ / ○ ◖▭◗	○ / ○	○ ◖▭◗ / ○	▭ / ▭
Sunday	○ ● ◖▭◗ / ○ ◖▭◗	○ / ○	○ ◖▭◗ / ○	▭ / ▭

Answer Form Station #1

MAR Answer Sheet

Identified mistake(s) or omission(s)	Rx1 (Drug1)	Rx2 (Drug2)	Rx3 (Drug 3)	Rx4 (Drug 4)
Drug				
Drug strength				
Drug dosage form				
Drug schedule				
Directions of use				
No problem				

Blister-Pack Answer Sheet

	Rx1 (Drug 1)				Rx2 (Drug 2)			
	AM	NOON	PM	HS	AM	NOON	PM	HS
Monday								
Tuesday								
Wednesday								
Thursday								
Friday								
Saturday								
Sunday								
	Rx3 (Drug 3)				Rx4 (Drug 4)			
	AM	NOON	PM	HS	AM	NOON	PM	HS
Monday								
Tuesday								
Wednesday								
Thursday								
Friday								
Saturday								
Sunday								

Answer Key Station #1

MAR Answer Key

Identified mistake(s) or omission(s)	Rx1 (Drug1)	Rx2 (Drug2)	Rx3 (Drug 3)	Rx4 (Drug 4)
Drug				• Xeloda tablets instead of Valcyte
Drug strength				
Drug dosage form				
Drug schedule		• Once a day		
Directions of use		• Once a day		
No problem	•		•	

Blister-Pack Answer Key

	Rx1 (Drug 1)				Rx2 (Drug 2)			
	AM	NOON	PM	HS	AM	NOON	PM	HS
Monday							•	
Tuesday			•				•	
Wednesday							•	
Thursday							•	
Friday			•				•	
Saturday							•	
Sunday							•	
	Rx3 (Drug 3)				Rx4 (Drug 4)			
	AM	NOON	PM	HS	AM	NOON	PM	HS
Monday								
Tuesday								
Wednesday								
Thursday								
Friday								
Saturday								
Sunday								

Non-interactive Station #2: Prescriptions/MAR/Blister-Pack Check

Candidate's instructions:

Check the accuracy of the Medication Administration Record (MAR) and Blister-Pack (see below) against the written prescriptions. Record **all** identified mistake(s) and omission(s) on the MAR and Blister-Pack answer form by filling the corresponding circle(s). You have a total of **4 prescriptions** in this station. <u>Note</u>: Make sure to check the shape and shade of tablets, and shade of capsules.

<u>This station must be completed in 6 minutes</u>

Written Prescriptions

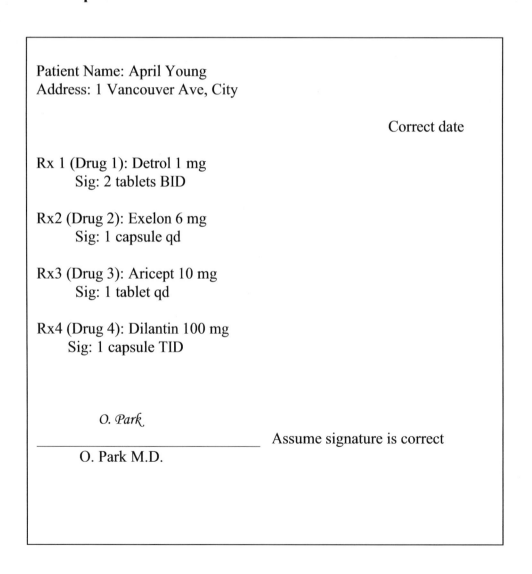

Patient Name: April Young
Address: 1 Vancouver Ave, City

Correct date

Rx 1 (Drug 1): Detrol 1 mg
    Sig: 2 tablets BID

Rx2 (Drug 2): Exelon 6 mg
    Sig: 1 capsule qd

Rx3 (Drug 3): Aricept 10 mg
    Sig: 1 tablet qd

Rx4 (Drug 4): Dilantin 100 mg
    Sig: 1 capsule TID

O. Park
_____   Assume signature is correct
    O. Park M.D.

Medication Administration Record (MAR)

Patient   April Young   **Date of birth**   November 3, 1945
Address   1 Vancouver Ave, City   **Gender**   Female
Phone   222-5555   **Allergies**   None known

Physician   Dr. O. Park
Address   First Road, City
Phone   888-7777

Medications	Description and dosage form	Directions of use	6 AM	NOON	6 PM	HS
Drug 1	Tablet, round white	2 tablets q12h	2			2
Drug 2	Tablet, elongated	1 tablet qd	1			
Drug 3	Tablet, round black	1 tablet qd	1			
Drug 4	Capsule	1 capsule TID	1	1	1	

Blister-Pack

Detrol ○   Exelon ◖   Aricept ●   Dilantin ◖

	AM	NOON	PM	HS
Monday	● ○ ◖ ○ ◖	◖	◖	○ ○
Tuesday	● ○ ◖ ○ ◖	◖ ◖	◖	○ ○
Wednesday	● ○ ◖ ○ ◖	◖	◖	○ ○
Thursday	● ○ ◖ ○ ◖	◖	◖	○ ○
Friday	● ○ ◖ ○ ◖	◖ ◖	◖	○ ○
Saturday	● ○ ◖ ○ ◖	◖	◖	○ ○
Sunday	● ○ ◖ ○ ◖	◖	◖ ◖	○ ○

Answer Form Station #2

MAR Answer Sheet

Identified mistake(s) or omission(s)	Rx1 (Drug1)	Rx2 (Drug2)	Rx3 (Drug 3)	Rx4 (Drug 4)
Drug				
Drug strength				
Drug dosage form				
Drug schedule				
Directions of use				
No problem				

Blister-Pack Answer Sheet

	Rx1 (Drug 1)				Rx2 (Drug 2)			
	AM	NOON	PM	HS	AM	NOON	PM	HS
Monday								
Tuesday								
Wednesday								
Thursday								
Friday								
Saturday								
Sunday								

	Rx3 (Drug 3)				Rx4 (Drug 4)			
	AM	NOON	PM	HS	AM	NOON	PM	HS
Monday								
Tuesday								
Wednesday								
Thursday								
Friday								
Saturday								
Sunday								

Answer Key Station #2

MAR Answer Key

Identified mistake(s) or omission(s)	Rx1 (Drug1)	Rx2 (Drug2)	Rx3 (Drug 3)	Rx4 (Drug 4)
Drug				
Drug strength				•
Drug dosage form		• Capsule not tablet		
Drug schedule	• Q12h not BID 6 PM instead of HS			
Directions of use				
No problem			•	

Blister-Pack Answer Key

	Rx1 (Drug 1)				Rx2 (Drug 2)			
	AM	NOON	PM	HS	AM	NOON	PM	HS
Monday			•	•				
Tuesday			•	•				
Wednesday			•	•				
Thursday			•	•				
Friday			•	•				
Saturday			•	•				
Sunday			•	•				
	Rx3 (Drug 3)				Rx4 (Drug 4)			
	AM	NOON	PM	HS	AM	NOON	PM	HS
Monday								
Tuesday						•		
Wednesday								
Thursday								
Friday						•		
Saturday								
Sunday							• 2 tabs not 1	

176

Non-interactive Station #3: Prescriptions/MAR/Blister-Pack Check

Candidate's instructions:

Check the accuracy of the Medication Administration Record (MAR) and Blister-Pack (see below) against the written prescriptions. Record **all** identified mistake(s) and omission(s) on the MAR and Blister-Pack answer form by filling the corresponding circle(s). You have a total of **4 prescriptions** in this station. <u>Note</u>: Make sure to check the shape and shade of tablets, and shade of capsules.

<u>This station must be completed in 6 minutes</u>

Written Prescriptions

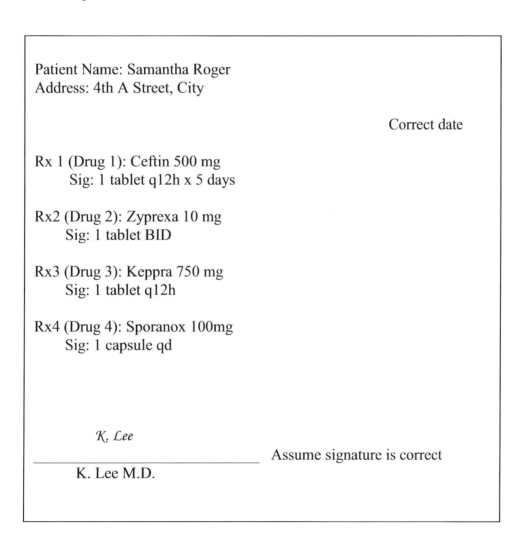

Patient Name: Samantha Roger
Address: 4th A Street, City

Correct date

Rx 1 (Drug 1): Ceftin 500 mg
    Sig: 1 tablet q12h x 5 days

Rx2 (Drug 2): Zyprexa 10 mg
    Sig: 1 tablet BID

Rx3 (Drug 3): Keppra 750 mg
    Sig: 1 tablet q12h

Rx4 (Drug 4): Sporanox 100mg
    Sig: 1 capsule qd

K. Lee
_____   Assume signature is correct
    K. Lee M.D.

Medication Administration Record (MAR)

Patient   Samantha Roger   **Date of birth**   June 14, 1970
Address   4th A Street, City   **Gender**   Female
Phone   111-1111   **Allergies**   None known

Physician   Dr. K. Lee
Address   88 Sunny St.
Phone   333-9999

Medications	Description and dosage form	Directions of use	6 AM	NOON	6 PM	HS
Drug 1	Tablet, white elongated	1 tablet q12h	1		1	
Drug 2	Tablet, round grey	1 tablet BID	1			1
Drug 3	Tablet, oval	1 tablet q12h	1		1	
Drug 4	Capsule	1 capsule qd			1	

Blister-Pack

Ceftin ⬭ Zyprexa ◯ Keppra ⬬ Sporanox ▰

	AM	NOON	PM	HS
Monday	⬭ ◯ ⬬	⬭	⬭ ▰	◯
Tuesday	⬭ ◯ ⬬	⬭	⬭ ⬬ ▰	◯
Wednesday	⬭ ◯ ⬬	⬭	⬭ ⬬ ▰	◯
Thursday	⬭ ◯ ⬬	⬭	⬭ ⬬ ▰	◯
Friday	⬭ ◯ ⬬	⬭	⬭ ⬬ ▰	◯
Saturday	⬭ ◯ ⬬	⬭	⬭ ⬬ ▰	◯
Sunday	⬭ ◯ ⬬	⬭	⬭ ▰	◯

Answer Form Station #3

MAR Answer Sheet

Identified mistake(s) or omission(s)	Rx1 (Drug1)	Rx2 (Drug2)	Rx3 (Drug 3)	Rx4 (Drug 4)
Drug				
Drug strength				
Drug dosage form				
Drug schedule				
Directions of use				
No problem				

Blister-Pack Answer Sheet

	Rx1 (Drug 1)				Rx2 (Drug 2)			
	AM	NOON	PM	HS	AM	NOON	PM	HS
Monday								
Tuesday								
Wednesday								
Thursday								
Friday								
Saturday								
Sunday								
	Rx3 (Drug 3)				Rx4 (Drug 4)			
	AM	NOON	PM	HS	AM	NOON	PM	HS
Monday								
Tuesday								
Wednesday								
Thursday								
Friday								
Saturday								
Sunday								

Answer Key Station #3

MAR Answer Key

Identified mistake(s) or omission(s)	Rx1 (Drug1)	Rx2 (Drug2)	Rx3 (Drug 3)	Rx4 (Drug 4)
Drug				
Drug strength				
Drug dosage form				
Drug schedule				
Directions of use				
No problem	●	●	●	●

Blister-Pack Answer Key

	Rx1 (Drug 1)				Rx2 (Drug 2)			
	AM	NOON	PM	HS	AM	NOON	PM	HS
Monday		●						
Tuesday		●						
Wednesday		●						
Thursday		●						
Friday		●						
Saturday	● For only 5 days	● Q12h not TID	●					
Sunday	●	●	●					

	Rx3 (Drug 3)				Rx4 (Drug 4)			
	AM	NOON	PM	HS	AM	NOON	PM	HS
Monday			●					
Tuesday								
Wednesday								
Thursday								
Friday								
Saturday								
Sunday			●					

Non-interactive Station #4: Prescriptions/MAR/Blister-Pack Check

Candidate's instructions:

Check the accuracy of the Medication Administration Record (MAR) and Blister-Pack (see below) against the written prescriptions. Record **all** identified mistake(s) and omission(s) on the MAR and Blister-Pack answer form by filling the corresponding circle(s). You have a total of **4 prescriptions** in this station. <u>Note</u>: Make sure to check the shape and shade of tablets, and shade of capsules.

<u>This station must be completed in 6 minutes</u>

Written Prescriptions

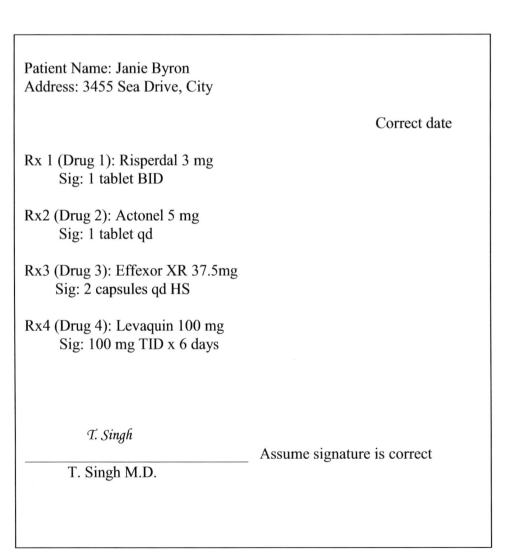

Patient Name: Janie Byron
Address: 3455 Sea Drive, City

Correct date

Rx 1 (Drug 1): Risperdal 3 mg
    Sig: 1 tablet BID

Rx2 (Drug 2): Actonel 5 mg
    Sig: 1 tablet qd

Rx3 (Drug 3): Effexor XR 37.5mg
    Sig: 2 capsules qd HS

Rx4 (Drug 4): Levaquin 100 mg
    Sig: 100 mg TID x 6 days

T. Singh
_____ Assume signature is correct
    T. Singh M.D.

Medication Administration Record (MAR)

Patient Janie Byron   **Date of birth** October 23, 1965
Address 3455 Drive, City   **Gender** Female
Phone 333-7878   **Allergies** None

Physician Dr. T. Singh
Address 1 Goodwill, City
Phone 666-6666

Medications	Description and dosage form	Directions of use	6 AM	NOON	6 PM	HS
Drug 1	Tablet, elongated with dots	1 tablet BID	1		1	
Drug 2	Tablet, elongated white	1 tablet qd	1		(1)	
Drug 3	Capsule	2 capsules qd HS	(2)			
Drug 4	Capsule	1 capsule TID	1	1	1	

Blister-Pack

Risperdal (··)   Actonel ⬭   Effexor ◖▭◗   Levaquin ⬬

	AM	NOON	PM	HS
Monday	(··) ⬬ ◖▭◗ ◖▭◗	⬬	⬭̸ ⬬ (··)	
Tuesday	(··) ⬬ ◖▭◗ ◖▭◗	⬬	⬭ ⬬ (··)	
Wednesday	(··) ⬬ ◖▭◗ ◖▭◗	⬬	⬭ ⬬ (··)	
Thursday	(··) ⬬ ◖▭◗ ◖▭◗	⬬	⬭ ⬬ (··)	
Friday	(··) ⬬ ◖▭◗ ◖▭◗	⬬	⬭ ⬬ (··)	
Saturday	(··) ⬬ ◖▭◗ ◖▭◗	⬬	⬭ ⬬ (··)	
Sunday	(··) ⬬̸ ◖▭◗ ◖▭◗	⬬̸	⬭ ⬬̸ (··)	

Answer Form Station #4

MAR Answer Sheet

Identified mistake(s) or omission(s)	Rx1 (Drug1)	Rx2 (Drug2)	Rx3 (Drug 3)	Rx4 (Drug 4)
Drug				
Drug strength				
Drug dosage form				
Drug schedule				
Directions of use				
No problem				

Blister-Pack Answer Sheet

	Rx1 (Drug 1)				Rx2 (Drug 2)			
	AM	NOON	PM	HS	AM	NOON	PM	HS
Monday								
Tuesday								
Wednesday								
Thursday								
Friday								
Saturday								
Sunday								

	Rx3 (Drug 3)				Rx4 (Drug 4)			
	AM	NOON	PM	HS	AM	NOON	PM	HS
Monday								
Tuesday								
Wednesday								
Thursday								
Friday								
Saturday								
Sunday								

Answer Key Station #4

MAR Answer Key

Identified mistake(s) or omission(s)	Rx1 (Drug1)	Rx2 (Drug2)	Rx3 (Drug 3)	Rx4 (Drug 4)
Drug				
Drug strength		● Need 5 mg not 30 mg		● 100 mg not 500 mg
Drug dosage form				●
Drug schedule		● qd not BID	● At bedtime	
Directions of use		●		
No problem	●			

Blister-Pack Answer Key

	Rx1 (Drug 1)				Rx2 (Drug 2)			
	AM	NOON	PM	HS	AM	NOON	PM	HS
Monday							•	
Tuesday							•	
Wednesday							•	
Thursday							•	
Friday							•	
Saturday							•	
Sunday							•	
	Rx3 (Drug 3)				Rx4 (Drug 4)			
	AM	NOON	PM	HS	AM	NOON	PM	HS
Monday	•			•				
Tuesday	•			•				
Wednesday	•			•				
Thursday	•			•				
Friday	•			•				
Saturday	•			•				
Sunday	•			•	•	• For only 6 days	•	

190

Non-interactive Station #5: Prescriptions/MAR/Blister-Pack Check

Candidate's instructions:

Check the accuracy of the Medication Administration Record (MAR) and Blister-Pack (see below) against the written prescriptions. Record **all** identified mistake(s) and omission(s) on the MAR and Blister-Pack answer form by filling the corresponding circle(s). You have a total of **4 prescriptions** in this station. Note: Make sure to check the shape and shade of tablets, and shade of capsules.

This station must be completed in 6 minutes

Written Prescriptions

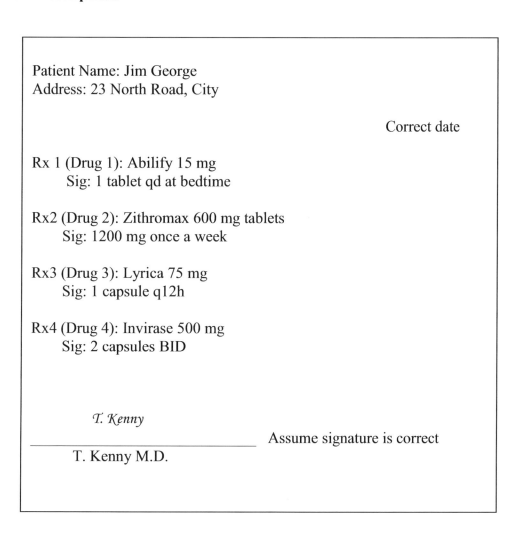

Patient Name: Jim George
Address: 23 North Road, City

Correct date

Rx 1 (Drug 1): Abilify 15 mg
    Sig: 1 tablet qd at bedtime

Rx2 (Drug 2): Zithromax 600 mg tablets
    Sig: 1200 mg once a week

Rx3 (Drug 3): Lyrica 75 mg
    Sig: 1 capsule q12h

Rx4 (Drug 4): Invirase 500 mg
    Sig: 2 capsules BID

T. Kenny
_____ Assume signature is correct
    T. Kenny M.D.

Medication Administration Record (MAR)

Patient   Jim George   **Date of birth**   March 7, 1975
Address   23 North Road, City   **Gender**   Male
Phone   999-8888   **Allergies**   None

Physician   Dr. T. Kenny
Address   4 Health St, City
Phone   555-6666

Medications	Description and dosage form	Directions of use	6 AM	NOON	6 PM	HS
Drug 1	Tablet, round	1 tablet qd HS				1
Drug 2	Tablet, elongated	2 tablets once a week	2			
Drug 3	Capsule	1 capsule q12h	1		1	
Drug 4	Capsule	2 capsules BID	2			2

Blister-Pack

Abilify ◯   Zithromax ⬭   Lyrica ⬲   Invirase ⬲

	AM	NOON	PM	HS
Monday	⬭ ⬲ ⬭ ⬲		⬲	◯ ⬲
Tuesday	⬭ ⬲ ⬭ ⬲		⬲	◯ ⬲
Wednesday	⬭ ⬲ ⬭ ⬲		⬲	◯ ⬲
Thursday	⬭ ⬲ ⬭ ⬲		⬲	◯ ⬲
Friday	⬭ ⬲ ⬭ ⬲		⬲	◯ ⬲
Saturday	⬭ ⬲ ⬭ ⬲		⬲	⬲
Sunday	⬭ ⬲ ⬭ ⬲		⬲	⬲

Answer Form Station #5

MAR Answer Sheet

Identified mistake(s) or omission(s)	Rx1 (Drug1)	Rx2 (Drug2)	Rx3 (Drug 3)	Rx4 (Drug 4)
Drug				
Drug strength				
Drug dosage form				
Drug schedule				
Directions of use				
No problem				

Blister-Pack Answer Sheet

	Rx1 (Drug 1)				Rx2 (Drug 2)			
	AM	NOON	PM	HS	AM	NOON	PM	HS
Monday								
Tuesday								
Wednesday								
Thursday								
Friday								
Saturday								
Sunday								
	Rx3 (Drug 3)				Rx4 (Drug 4)			
	AM	NOON	PM	HS	AM	NOON	PM	HS
Monday								
Tuesday								
Wednesday								
Thursday								
Friday								
Saturday								
Sunday								

Answer Key Station #5

MAR Answer Key

Identified mistake(s) or omission(s)	Rx1 (Drug1)	Rx2 (Drug2)	Rx3 (Drug 3)	Rx4 (Drug 4)
Drug				
Drug strength				● 500 mg needed not 200 mg
Drug dosage form				
Drug schedule				
Directions of use				
No problem	●	●	●	

Blister-Pack Answer Key

	Rx1 (Drug 1)				Rx2 (Drug 2)			
	AM	NOON	PM	HS	AM	NOON	PM	HS
Monday								
Tuesday					• 2 tabs per wk			
Wednesday					•			
Thursday					•			
Friday					•			
Saturday				• Missing tab	•			
Sunday				•	•			

	Rx3 (Drug 3)				Rx4 (Drug 4)			
	AM	NOON	PM	HS	AM	NOON	PM	HS
Monday					• 2 caps not 1			•
Tuesday					•			•
Wednesday					•			•
Thursday					•			•
Friday					•			•
Saturday					•			•
Sunday					•			•

Non-interactive Station #6: Prescriptions/MAR/Blister-Pack Check

Candidate's instructions:

Check the accuracy of the Medication Administration Record (MAR) and Blister-Pack (see below) against the written prescriptions. Record **all** identified mistake(s) and omission(s) on the MAR and Blister-Pack answer form by filling the corresponding circle(s). You have a total of **4 prescriptions** in this station. <u>Note</u>: Make sure to check the shape and shade of tablets, and shade of capsules.

<u>This station must be completed in 6 minutes</u>

Written Prescriptions

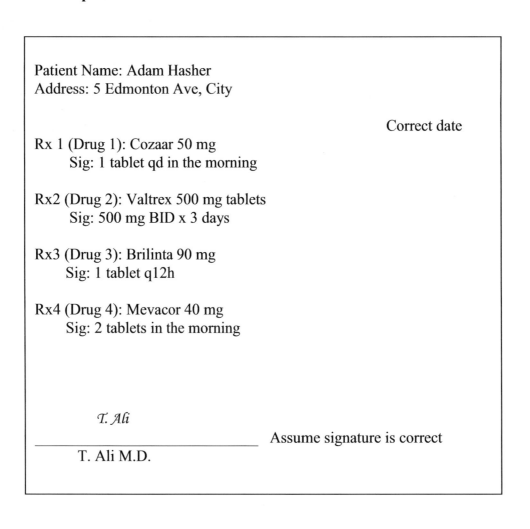

Patient Name: Adam Hasher
Address: 5 Edmonton Ave, City

Correct date

Rx 1 (Drug 1): Cozaar 50 mg
    Sig: 1 tablet qd in the morning

Rx2 (Drug 2): Valtrex 500 mg tablets
    Sig: 500 mg BID x 3 days

Rx3 (Drug 3): Brilinta 90 mg
    Sig: 1 tablet q12h

Rx4 (Drug 4): Mevacor 40 mg
    Sig: 2 tablets in the morning

T. Ali
_____   Assume signature is correct
    T. Ali M.D.

Medication Administration Record (MAR)

Patient	Adam Hasher	**Date of birth**	April 1, 1960
Address	5 Edm Ave, City	**Gender**	Male
Phone	444-0000	**Allergies**	None

Physician	Dr. T. Ali
Address	Sunny Square, City
Phone	101-1010

Medications	Description and dosage form	Directions of use	6 AM	NOON	6 PM	HS
Drug 1	Tablet, oval white	1 tablet qd AM	1			
Drug 2	Capsule with dots	1 capsule BID	1		1	
Drug 3	Capsule with 1 dot	1 capsule q12h	1		1	
Drug 4	Tablet, round	2 tablets HS	2			

Blister-Pack

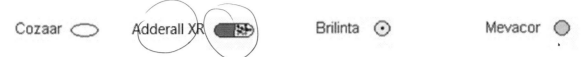

Cozaar ⬭   Adderall XR 🔴   Brilinta ⊙   Mevacor ⚪

	AM	NOON	PM	HS
Monday	◯ ◯ ⊙ ⬭ 🔴		⊙ 🔴	⬭
Tuesday	◯ ◯ ⊙ ⬭ 🔴		⊙ 🔴	⬭
Wednesday	◯ ◯ ⊙ ⬭ 🔴		⊙ 🔴	⬭
Thursday	◯ ◯ ⊙ ⬭ 🔴		⊙ 🔴	⬭
Friday	◯ ◯ ⊙ ⬭ 🔴		⊙ 🔴	⬭
Saturday	◯ ◯ ⊙ ⬭ 🔴		⊙ 🔴	⬭
Sunday	◯ ◯ ⊙ ⬭ 🔴		⊙ 🔴	⬭

Answer Form Station #6

MAR Answer Sheet

Identified mistake(s) or omission(s)	Rx1 (Drug1)	Rx2 (Drug2)	Rx3 (Drug 3)	Rx4 (Drug 4)
Drug				
Drug strength				
Drug dosage form				
Drug schedule				
Directions of use				
No problem				

Blister-Pack Answer Sheet

	Rx1 (Drug 1)				Rx2 (Drug 2)			
	AM	NOON	PM	HS	AM	NOON	PM	HS
Monday								
Tuesday								
Wednesday								
Thursday								
Friday								
Saturday								
Sunday								

	Rx3 (Drug 3)				Rx4 (Drug 4)			
	AM	NOON	PM	HS	AM	NOON	PM	HS
Monday								
Tuesday								
Wednesday								
Thursday								
Friday								
Saturday								
Sunday								

Answer Key Station #6

MAR Answer Key

Identified mistake(s) or omission(s)	Rx1 (Drug1)	Rx2 (Drug2)	Rx3 (Drug 3)	Rx4 (Drug 4)
Drug		● Adderall XR instead of Valtrex		
Drug strength				
Drug dosage form			● Tablet not capsule	
Drug schedule				● AM not HS
Directions of use				
No problem	●			

Blister-Pack Answer Key

	Rx1 (Drug 1)				Rx2 (Drug 2)			
	AM	NOON	PM	HS	AM	NOON	PM	HS
Monday				• qd not bid				
Tuesday				•				
Wednesday				•				
Thursday				•	• For only 3 days		•	
Friday				•	•		•	
Saturday				•	•		•	
Sunday				•	•		•	

	Rx3 (Drug 3)				Rx4 (Drug 4)			
	AM	NOON	PM	HS	AM	NOON	PM	HS
Monday								
Tuesday								
Wednesday								
Thursday								
Friday								
Saturday								
Sunday								

Non-interactive Station #7: Prescriptions/MAR/Blister-Pack Check

Candidate's instructions:

Check the accuracy of the Medication Administration Record (MAR) and Blister-Pack (see below) against the written prescriptions. Record **all** identified mistake(s) and omission(s) on the MAR and Blister-Pack answer form by filling the corresponding circle(s). You have a total of **4 prescriptions** in this station. <u>Note</u>: Make sure to check the shape and shade of tablets, and shade of capsules.

<u>This station must be completed in 6 minutes</u>

Written Prescriptions

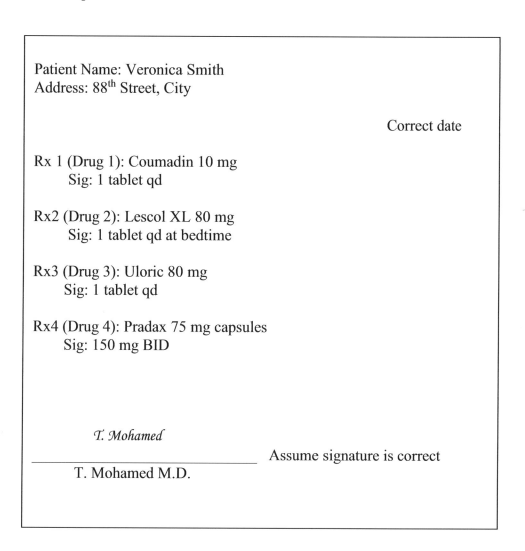

Patient Name: Veronica Smith
Address: 88th Street, City

Correct date

Rx 1 (Drug 1): Coumadin 10 mg
    Sig: 1 tablet qd

Rx2 (Drug 2): Lescol XL 80 mg
    Sig: 1 tablet qd at bedtime

Rx3 (Drug 3): Uloric 80 mg
    Sig: 1 tablet qd

Rx4 (Drug 4): Pradax 75 mg capsules
    Sig: 150 mg BID

T. Mohamed
_____ Assume signature is correct
    T. Mohamed M.D.

Medication Administration Record (MAR)

Patient	Veronica Smith	Date of birth	December 15, 1947
Address	88th Street, City	Gender	Female
Phone	222-3333	Allergies	None

Physician	Dr. T. Mohamed
Address	1A Hospital Rd
Phone	200-0000

Medications	Description and dosage form	Directions of use	6 AM	NOON	6 PM	HS
Drug 1	Tablet, round white	1 tablet qd	1			
Drug 2	Tablet, round dark	1 tablet qd HS				1
Drug 3	Tablet, oval	1 tablet qd	1			
Drug 4	Capsule	2 capsules TID	2	2		2

Blister-Pack

Coumadin ○   Lescol XL ●   Uloric ⬬   Pradax ◖▭

	AM	NOON	PM	HS
Monday	◖▭ ◖▭ ⬬ ○	◖▭ ◖▭		◖▭ ◖▭
Tuesday	◖▭ ◖▭ ⬬ ○	◖▭ ◖▭		◖▭
Wednesday	◖▭ ◖▭ ⬬ ○	◖▭ ◖▭		◖▭
Thursday	◖▭ ◖▭ ⬬ ○	◖▭ ◖▭		◖▭ ◖▭
Friday	◖▭ ◖▭ ⬬ ○	◖▭ ◖▭		◖▭ ◖▭
Saturday	◖▭ ◖▭ ⬬ ○	◖▭ ◖▭		◖▭ ◖▭
Sunday	◖▭ ◖▭ ⬬ ○	◖▭ ◖▭		◖▭ ◖▭

207

Answer Form Station #7

MAR Answer Sheet

Identified mistake(s) or omission(s)	Rx1 (Drug1)	Rx2 (Drug2)	Rx3 (Drug 3)	Rx4 (Drug 4)
Drug				
Drug strength				
Drug dosage form				
Drug schedule				
Directions of use				
No problem				

Blister-Pack Answer Sheet

	Rx1 (Drug 1)				Rx2 (Drug 2)			
	AM	NOON	PM	HS	AM	NOON	PM	HS
Monday								
Tuesday								
Wednesday								
Thursday								
Friday								
Saturday								
Sunday								

	Rx3 (Drug 3)				Rx4 (Drug 4)			
	AM	NOON	PM	HS	AM	NOON	PM	HS
Monday								
Tuesday								
Wednesday								
Thursday								
Friday								
Saturday								
Sunday								

Answer Key Station #7

MAR Answer Key

Identified mistake(s) or omission(s)	Rx1 (Drug1)	Rx2 (Drug2)	Rx3 (Drug 3)	Rx4 (Drug 4)
Drug				
Drug strength				
Drug dosage form				
Drug schedule				•
Directions of use				• BID not TID
No problem	•	•	•	

Blister-Pack Answer Key

	Rx1 (Drug 1)				Rx2 (Drug 2)			
	AM	NOON	PM	HS	AM	NOON	PM	HS
Monday								• Missing pill
Tuesday								•
Wednesday								•
Thursday								•
Friday								•
Saturday								•
Sunday								•

	Rx3 (Drug 3)				Rx4 (Drug 4)			
	AM	NOON	PM	HS	AM	NOON	PM	HS
Monday						•		
Tuesday						•		
Wednesday						•		
Thursday						•		
Friday						•		
Saturday						•		
Sunday						•		

Non-interactive Station #8: Prescriptions/MAR/Blister-Pack Check

Candidate's instructions:

Check the accuracy of the Medication Administration Record (MAR) and Blister-Pack (see below) against the written prescriptions. Record **all** identified mistake(s) and omission(s) on the MAR and Blister-Pack answer form by filling the corresponding circle(s). You have a total of **4 prescriptions** in this station. <u>Note</u>: Make sure to check the shape and shade of tablets, and shade of capsules.

<u>This station must be completed in 6 minutes</u>

Written Prescriptions

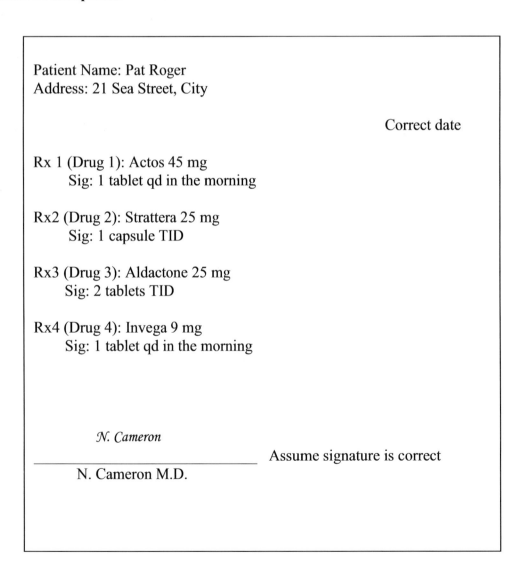

Patient Name: Pat Roger
Address: 21 Sea Street, City

Correct date

Rx 1 (Drug 1): Actos 45 mg
    Sig: 1 tablet qd in the morning

Rx2 (Drug 2): Strattera 25 mg
    Sig: 1 capsule TID

Rx3 (Drug 3): Aldactone 25 mg
    Sig: 2 tablets TID

Rx4 (Drug 4): Invega 9 mg
    Sig: 1 tablet qd in the morning

N. Cameron
_____ Assume signature is correct
    N. Cameron M.D.

Medication Administration Record (MAR)

Patient   Pat Roger   **Date of birth**   July 6, 1966

Address   21 Sea Street, City   **Gender**   Male

Phone   505-5555   **Allergies**   None

Physician   Dr. N. Cameron

Address   5T Blue St., City

Phone   999-1010

Medications	Description and dosage form	Directions of use	6 AM	NOON	6 PM	HS
Drug 1	Tablet, round white	1 tablet qd AM	1			
Drug 2	Tablet, elongated	1 tablet TID	1	1	1	
Drug 3	Tablet, round dark	2 tablets TID	2	2	2	
Drug 4	Tablet, rectangular	1 tablet qd AM	1			

Blister-Pack

Actos ○   Strattera ⬭   Aldactone ⬤   Invega ▭

	AM	NOON	PM	HS
Monday	▭ ● ⬭ ●	⬭ ●	⬭ ● ●	○
Tuesday	▭ ● ⬭ ●	⬭ ●	⬭ ● ●	○
Wednesday	● ▭ ●	⬭ ●	⬭ ● ●	○ ▭
Thursday	▭ ● ⬭ ●	⬭ ● ●	⬭ ● ●	○
Friday	▭ ● ⬭ ●	⬭ ● ●	⬭ ● ●	○
Saturday	● ⬭ ●	⬭ ● ●	⬭ ● ●	○ ▭
Sunday	▭ ● ⬭ ●	⬭ ●	⬭ ● ●	○

214

Answer Form Station #8

MAR Answer Sheet

Identified mistake(s) or omission(s)	Rx1 (Drug1)	Rx2 (Drug2)	Rx3 (Drug 3)	Rx4 (Drug 4)
Drug				
Drug strength				
Drug dosage form				
Drug schedule				
Directions of use				
No problem				

Blister-Pack Answer Sheet

	Rx1 (Drug 1)				Rx2 (Drug 2)			
	AM	NOON	PM	HS	AM	NOON	PM	HS
Monday								
Tuesday								
Wednesday								
Thursday								
Friday								
Saturday								
Sunday								

	Rx3 (Drug 3)				Rx4 (Drug 4)			
	AM	NOON	PM	HS	AM	NOON	PM	HS
Monday								
Tuesday								
Wednesday								
Thursday								
Friday								
Saturday								
Sunday								

Answer Key Station #8

MAR Answer Key

Identified mistake(s) or omission(s)	Rx1 (Drug1)	Rx2 (Drug2)	Rx3 (Drug 3)	Rx4 (Drug 4)
Drug				
Drug strength				
Drug dosage form		● Capsule not tablet		
Drug schedule				
Directions of use				
No problem	●			●

Blister-Pack Answer Key

	Rx1 (Drug 1)				Rx2 (Drug 2)			
	AM	NOON	PM	HS	AM	NOON	PM	HS
Monday	•			•				
Tuesday	•			•				
Wednesday	•			•				
Thursday	•			•				
Friday	•			•				
Saturday	•			•				
Sunday	•			•				
	Rx3 (Drug 3)				Rx4 (Drug 4)			
	AM	NOON	PM	HS	AM	NOON	PM	HS
Monday		•						
Tuesday		•						
Wednesday		• Missing pill			•			•
Thursday								
Friday								
Saturday					•			•
Sunday		•						

Non-interactive Station #9: Prescriptions/MAR/Blister-Pack Check

Candidate's instructions:

Check the accuracy of the Medication Administration Record (MAR) and Blister-Pack (see below) against the written prescriptions. Record **all** identified mistake(s) and omission(s) on the MAR and Blister-Pack answer form by filling the corresponding circle(s). You have a total of **4 prescriptions** in this station. <u>Note</u>: Make sure to check the shape and shade of tablets, and shade of capsules.

<u>This station must be completed in 6 minutes</u>

Written Prescriptions

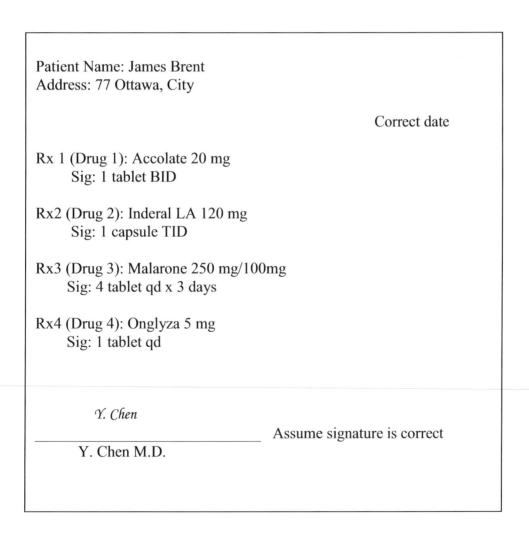

Patient Name: James Brent
Address: 77 Ottawa, City

Correct date

Rx 1 (Drug 1): Accolate 20 mg
    Sig: 1 tablet BID

Rx2 (Drug 2): Inderal LA 120 mg
    Sig: 1 capsule TID

Rx3 (Drug 3): Malarone 250 mg/100mg
    Sig: 4 tablet qd x 3 days

Rx4 (Drug 4): Onglyza 5 mg
    Sig: 1 tablet qd

Y. Chen
_____   Assume signature is correct
    Y. Chen M.D.

Medication Administration Record (MAR)

Patient	James Brent	**Date of birth**	April 8, 1968
Address	77 Ottawa, City	**Gender**	Male
Phone	666-0777	**Allergies**	None

Physician	Dr. Y. Chen
Address	8 Spring Drive
Phone	333-9090

Medications	Description and dosage form	Directions of use	6 AM	NOON	6 PM	HS
Drug 1	Tablet, round white	1 tablet BID	1		1	
Drug 2	Capsule	1 capsule TID	1	1	1	
Drug 3	Tablet, round dark	4 tablets qd	4			
Drug 4	Tablet, round with 1 dot	1 tablet qd	1			

Blister-Pack

Accolate ○   Inderal LA ▭   Malarone ●   Onglyza ◉

	AM	NOON	PM	HS
Monday	● ● ▭ ● ◉ ● ○	▭	○ ▭	○
Tuesday	● ● ▭ ● ◉ ● ○	▭	○ ▭	○ ◉
Wednesday	● ● ▭ ● ◉ ○	▭	○ ▭	○
Thursday	▭ ◉ ○	▭	○	○ ◉
Friday	▭ ◉ ○	▭	○	○
Saturday	▭ ◉ ○	▭	○ ▭	○ ◉
Sunday	◉ ○	▭	○ ▭	○

Answer Form Station #9

MAR Answer Sheet

Identified mistake(s) or omission(s)	Rx1 (Drug1)	Rx2 (Drug2)	Rx3 (Drug 3)	Rx4 (Drug 4)
Drug				
Drug strength				
Drug dosage form				
Drug schedule				
Directions of use				
No problem				

Blister-Pack Answer Sheet

	Rx1 (Drug 1)				Rx2 (Drug 2)			
	AM	NOON	PM	HS	AM	NOON	PM	HS
Monday								
Tuesday								
Wednesday								
Thursday								
Friday								
Saturday								
Sunday								
	Rx3 (Drug 3)				Rx4 (Drug 4)			
	AM	NOON	PM	HS	AM	NOON	PM	HS
Monday								
Tuesday								
Wednesday								
Thursday								
Friday								
Saturday								
Sunday								

Answer Key Station #9

MAR Answer Key

Identified mistake(s) or omission(s)	Rx1 (Drug1)	Rx2 (Drug2)	Rx3 (Drug 3)	Rx4 (Drug 4)
Drug				
Drug strength				
Drug dosage form				
Drug schedule				
Directions of use				
No problem	●	●	●	●

Blister-Pack Answer Key

	Rx1 (Drug 1)				Rx2 (Drug 2)			
	AM	NOON	PM	HS	AM	NOON	PM	HS
Monday				• Extra pill				
Tuesday				•				
Wednesday				•				
Thursday				•			• Missing pill	
Friday				•			•	
Saturday				•				
Sunday				•	• Missing pill			

	Rx3 (Drug 3)				Rx4 (Drug 4)			
	AM	NOON	PM	HS	AM	NOON	PM	HS
Monday								
Tuesday								• Extra pill
Wednesday	• Missing pill							
Thursday								•
Friday								
Saturday								•
Sunday								

Non-interactive Station #10: Prescriptions/MAR/Blister-Pack Check

Candidate's instructions:

Check the accuracy of the Medication Administration Record (MAR) and Blister-Pack (see below) against the written prescriptions. Record **all** identified mistake(s) and omission(s) on the MAR and Blister-Pack answer form by filling the corresponding circle(s). You have a total of **4 prescriptions** in this station. <u>Note</u>: Make sure to check the shape and shade of tablets, and shade of capsules.

<u>This station must be completed in 6 minutes</u>

Written Prescriptions

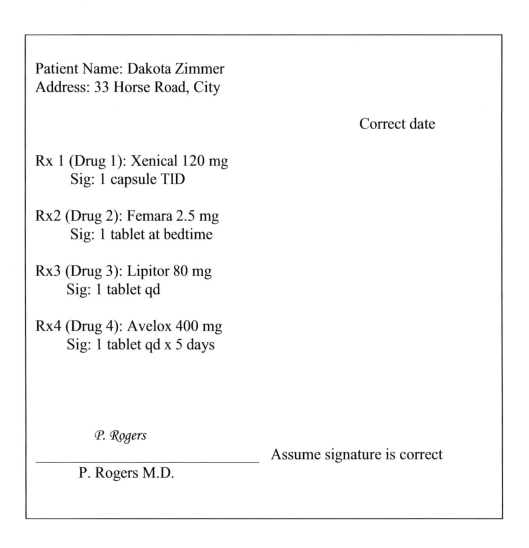

Patient Name: Dakota Zimmer
Address: 33 Horse Road, City

Correct date

Rx 1 (Drug 1): Xenical 120 mg
    Sig: 1 capsule TID

Rx2 (Drug 2): Femara 2.5 mg
    Sig: 1 tablet at bedtime

Rx3 (Drug 3): Lipitor 80 mg
    Sig: 1 tablet qd

Rx4 (Drug 4): Avelox 400 mg
    Sig: 1 tablet qd x 5 days

P. Rogers

_____ Assume signature is correct
    P. Rogers M.D.

Medication Administration Record (MAR)

Patient	Dakota Zimmer	**Date of birth**	August 25, 1962			
Address	33 Horse Road, City	**Gender**	Female			
Phone	233-7777	**Allergies**	None			

Physician Dr. P. Rogers
Address 5 Clinic Square, City
Phone 888-4545

Medications	Description and dosage form	Directions of use	6 AM	NOON	6 PM	HS
Drug 1	Capsule	1 capsule TID	1	1	1	
Drug 2	Capsule	1 capsule qd HS				1
Drug 3	Tablet, oval white	1 tablet qid	1	1	1	1
Drug 4	Tablet, elongated	1 tablet qd	1			

Blister-Pack

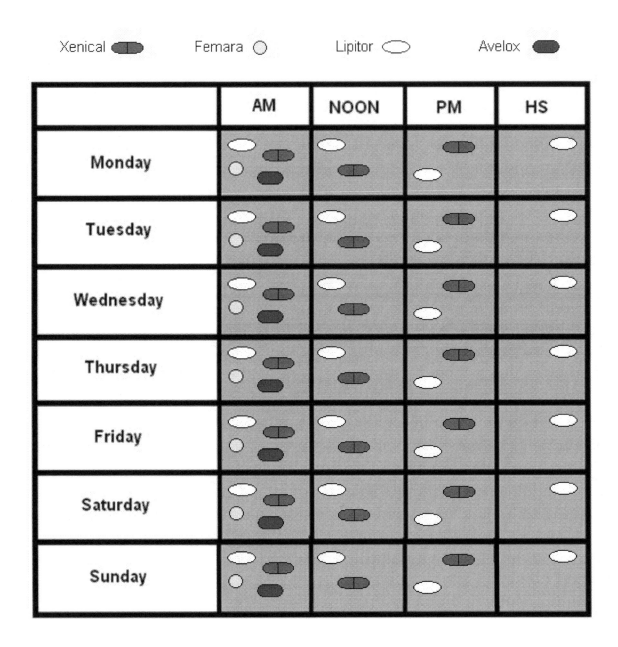

Answer Form Station #10

MAR Answer Sheet

Identified mistake(s) or omission(s)	Rx1 (Drug1)	Rx2 (Drug2)	Rx3 (Drug 3)	Rx4 (Drug 4)
Drug				
Drug strength				
Drug dosage form				
Drug schedule				
Directions of use				
No problem				

Blister-Pack Answer Sheet

	Rx1 (Drug 1)				Rx2 (Drug 2)			
	AM	NOON	PM	HS	AM	NOON	PM	HS
Monday								
Tuesday								
Wednesday								
Thursday								
Friday								
Saturday								
Sunday								

	Rx3 (Drug 3)				Rx4 (Drug 4)			
	AM	NOON	PM	HS	AM	NOON	PM	HS
Monday								
Tuesday								
Wednesday								
Thursday								
Friday								
Saturday								
Sunday								

Answer Key Station #10

MAR Answer Key

Identified mistake(s) or omission(s)	Rx1 (Drug1)	Rx2 (Drug2)	Rx3 (Drug 3)	Rx4 (Drug 4)
Drug				
Drug strength				
Drug dosage form		• Tablet not capsule		
Drug schedule			• qd not qid	
Directions of use			•	
No problem	•			•

Blister-Pack Answer Key

	Rx1 (Drug 1)				Rx2 (Drug 2)			
	AM	NOON	PM	HS	AM	NOON	PM	HS
Monday					•			•
Tuesday					•			•
Wednesday					•			•
Thursday					•			•
Friday					•			•
Saturday					•			•
Sunday					•			•

	Rx3 (Drug 3)				Rx4 (Drug 4)			
	AM	NOON	PM	HS	AM	NOON	PM	HS
Monday		•	•	•				
Tuesday		•	•	•				
Wednesday		•	•	•				
Thursday		•	•	•				
Friday		•	•	•				
Saturday		•	•	•	• For only 5 days			
Sunday		•	•	•	•			

OSPE Technical Skills Stations

Station #1: Sterile garbing and gowning skills

You are an experienced pharmacy technician responsible for training newly hired pharmacy technicians. Today, the pharmacy technician in training is showing you his sterile gowning skills. He is performing all required sterile garbing and gowning steps. You are expected to evaluate his performance at each step according to USP standards. Use the **answer form** to record your findings by filling the circles. If applicable, identify errors/omissions and order the steps accurately. <u>You have 6 minutes to complete this station.</u>

While you are watching, the pharmacy technician in training performed the following steps:

Step 1: He removes his coat, sweater, watch leaving a small wedding ring; his fingernails are short and neat.

Step 2: He puts on the following items: shoe covers, head cover enclosing his hair entirely, and face mask covering his mouth entirely leaving only his nose out to ease breathing.

Step 3: He performs the following hand cleansing procedure. He uses a nail cleaner under running warm water to remove debris from underneath fingernails followed by vigorous hand washing. He washes his hands and forearms to the elbows for at least 30 seconds with soap and warm water. He then dries completely his hands and forearms using an electronic hand dryer.

Step 4: He enters the cleanroom.

Step 5: He puts on a non-shedding disposable gown with sleeves that fit snugly around the wrists and enclosed at the neck.

Step 6: He then cleans his hands using a waterless alcohol-based hand scrub. He allows his hands to dry completely before donning sterile compounding gloves.

Step 7: He puts on sterile compounding gloves touching only the inner surface and non-sterile wrapper. He then inspects gloved hands for holes, punctures, or tears in gloves. He removes powder from gloves with alcohol spray. He clasps his hands together to avoid touching any surface then proceeds with compounding.

Answer Form - Compounding Skills Case #1

Procedures	Done accurately	Done incorrectly	Errors/omissions	Order the steps accurately
Step 1	O	O		
Step 2	O	O		
Step 3	O	O		
Step 4	O	O		
Step 5	O	O		
Step 6	O	O		
Step 7	O	O		

Answer Key – Compounding Skills Case #1

Procedures	Done accurately	Done incorrectly	Errors/omissions	Order the steps accurately
Step 1	O	●	The wedding ring must be removed	Step 1
Step 2	O	●	Nose and mouth must be covered	Step 2
Step 3	●	O	An electronic hand dryer can be used instead of a lint-free towel	Step 3
Step 4	●	O	The order is wrong. His gown must be on prior to entering the cleanroom	Step 5
Step 5	●	O	The order is wrong but the procedure is accurate	Step 4
Step 6	●	O		Step 6
Step 7	●	O	Hands must be allowed to dry; do not clasp hands	Step 7

Station #2: Sterile garbing and gowning skills

You are an experienced pharmacy technician responsible for training newly hired pharmacy technicians. Today, the pharmacy technician in training is showing you her sterile gowning skills. She is performing all required sterile garbing and gowning steps. You are expected to evaluate her performance at each step according to USP standards. Use the **answer form** to record your findings by filling the circles. If applicable, identify errors/omissions and order the steps accurately. You have 6 minutes to complete this station.

While you are watching, the pharmacy technician in training performed the following steps:

Step 1: She puts on the following items: shoe covers, head cover enclosing her hair entirely including her short pony tail, and face mask covering her mouth and nose.
Step 2: She removes her jacket, watch, two rings, one bracelet; she is not wearing make up and her fingernails are short and neat free of artificial nails.
Step 3: She enters the cleanroom.

Step 4: She performs the following hand cleansing procedure. She washes her hands to the wrist including underneath fingernails for at least 30 seconds with soap and warm water. She then dries completely her hands and forearms using a lint-free disposable towel then turns off tap with towel.

Step 5: She puts on a non-shedding reusable gown with sleeves that fit snugly around the wrists and enclosed at the neck.

Step 6: She then cleans her hands using a waterless alcohol-based hand scrub. She allows her hands to dry thoroughly before donning sterile compounding gloves.

Step 7: She puts on sterile compounding gloves touching the outer surface of gloves. She then inspects gloved hands for holes, punctures, or tears in gloves. She then proceeds with compounding.

Answer Form - Compounding Skills Case #2

Procedures	Done accurately	Done incorrectly	Errors/omissions	Order the steps accurately
Step 1	O	O		
Step 2	O	O		
Step 3	O	O		
Step 4	O	⊙		
Step 5	O	O		
Step 6	O	O		
Step 7	O	⊙	Touch only the inner surface	

Answer Key – Compounding Skills Case#2

Procedures	Done accurately	Done incorrectly	Errors/omissions	Order the steps accurately
Step 1	●	O	Wrong order but done accurately.	Step 2
Step 2	●	O	Wrong order but done accurately.	Step 1
Step 3	●	O	Wrong order	Step 5
Step 4	O	●	Must wash hands up to forearms and nails have not been scrubbed. Not enough scrubbing.	Step 3
Step 5	●	O		Step 4
Step 6	●	O		Step 6
Step 7	O	●	Must touch only the inner surface of gloves and non-sterile wrapper. He did not remove powder from gloves with alcohol spray.	Step 7

Station #3: Laminar Air Flow Cleaning/Items Placement/Working with Vials

You are an experienced pharmacy technician responsible for training newly hired pharmacy technicians. Today, the pharmacy technician in training is demonstrating her horizontal laminar air flow hood cleaning, items placement and working with vials skills. You are expected to evaluate her performance at each step according to USP standards. Use the **answer form** to record your findings by filling the circles. If applicable, identify errors/omissions and order the steps accurately. You have 6 minutes to complete this station.

While you are watching, the pharmacy technician in training performed the following steps:

Step 1: She uses a lint-free towel moistened with 70% isopropyl alcohol starting at the back of the hood in front of the HEPA filter and move horizontally from side to side and from back to front of the hood.

Step 2: She repeats step 1 using a fresh lint-free towel moistened with 70% alcohol. At each step she makes sure not to allow alcohol to make contact with the filter.

Step 3: She then turns the hood on and allows the hood to run for 45 minutes.

Step 4: She places two vials in the hood, one in front of the other, according to the order they will be used. She then sprays each vial with 70% isopropyl alcohol. She also places in the hood a wrapped sterile syringe and wrapped sterile needle, side by side separated by at least 3 inches.

Step 5: She works 6 inches from the front of the hood to avoid disruption of airflow. With her hands behind the vials, she swabs the rubber top of the first vial with alcohol swab using firm strokes in a unidirectional sweeping motion at least 3 times. She allows the alcohol to dry.

Step 6: She tears the sterile syringe wrapper and needle wrapper. She holds the tip of the syringe to attach the needle; she ensures not to touch any part of the needle.

Step 7: She then inserts the bevel tip of the needle first in the rubber top of the vial, then press downward and toward the bevel so that the bevel tip and heel enter at the same point. She proceeds to transfer appropriately the solution in the second vial.

Answer Form - Compounding Skills Case #3

Procedures	Done accurately	Done incorrectly	Errors/omissions	Order the steps accurately
Step 1	O	O		
Step 2	O	O		
Step 3	O	O		
Step 4	O	Ⓞ	vials placed side by side not behind, vials must be sprayed before entering ⚠️	
Step 5	O	Ⓞ	hands not behind the vial	
Step 6	O	Ⓞ	must be pealed not teared, don't touch syringe tip	
Step 7	O	O		

Answer Key - Compounding Skills Case #3

Procedures	Done accurately	Done incorrectly	Errors/omissions	Order the steps accurately
Step 1	●	O	Accurate but wrong order	Step 2
Step 2	●	O	Accurate but wrong order	Step 3
Step 3	●	O	Accurate but wrong order	Step 1
Step 4	O	●	Wrong vials placement; air flow is blocked by placing the vials one in front the other. They must be side by side. The vials must be sprayed with alcohol outside the hood.	Step 4
Step 5	O	●	By placing her hands behind the vials, airflow will be blocked and aseptic technique will be broken	Step 5
Step 6	O	●	Wrapper must be peeled; tearing releases particles The syringe tip and plunger must not be touched	Step 6
Step 7	●	O		Step 7

Station #4: Working with Ampules in the Laminar Air Flow Hood

You are an experienced pharmacy technician responsible for training newly hired pharmacy technicians. Today, the pharmacy technician in training is demonstrating how to break an ampule, withdraw and transfer a sample of the solution using a syringe under a horizontal laminar air hood. You are expected to evaluate his performance at each step according to USP standards. Use the **answer form** to record your findings by filling the circles. If applicable, identify errors/omissions and order the steps accurately. You have 6 minutes to complete this station.

While you are watching, the pharmacy technician in training performed the following steps:

Step 1: He swabs the neck of the ampule with an alcohol swab. Holds the ampule upright and tap the top to settle the solution into the ampule.

Step 2: He covers the ampule with a sterile gauze pad to protect his fingers. He aligns the thumbnails toward the desired point of breakage then applies quick and even pressure and snaps the ampule at the neck towards the filter. He discards the gauze and the severed portion of the ampule.

Step 3: He peels off the wrappers of a sterile syringe and sterile needle. He attaches the needle to the syringe ensuring not to touch any part of the needle nor the tip and plunger of the syringe.

Step 4: To withdraw the solution, he tilts the ampule at about a 20 degree angle, inserts the needle in the ampule without touching the opening then pulls back on syringe plunger. He keeps the needle submerged to avoid withdrawing air into the syringe.

Step 5: He removes the needle from ampule and removes all air bubbles from syringe, bringing it to final desired volume.

Step 6: He then uses his thumb the apply pressure on the syringe plunger to transfer the solution in a sterile container.

Step 7: He finally inspects the transferred solution for precipitation or other particulate matters.

Answer Form - Compounding Skills Case #4

Procedures	Done accurately	Done incorrectly	Errors/omissions	Order the steps accurately
Step 1	O	O		
Step 2	O	O		
Step 3	O	O		
Step 4	O	O		
Step 5	O	O		
Step 6	O	O		
Step 7	O	O		

Answer Key - Compounding Skills Case #4

Procedures	Done accurately	Done incorrectly	Errors/omissions	Order the steps accurately
Step 1	●	O		Step 1
Step 2	●	O		Step 2
Step 3	●	O		Step 3
Step 4	●	O		Step 4
Step 5	●	O		Step 5
Step 6	O	●	A filter needle must be used to complete the transfer of the solution into the sterile container; by using a filter needle potential glass particles are removed.	Step 6
Step 7	●	O		Step 7

Station #5: Preparation of an oral suspension

You are an experienced pharmacy technician responsible for training newly hired pharmacy technicians. Today, the pharmacy technician in training is demonstrating her compounding skills. She is preparing an oral suspension of aluminum hydroxide antacid according to the formula below. You are expected to evaluate her performance at each step. Use the **answer form** to record your findings by filling the circles and order the steps accurately if needed; if applicable identify errors/omissions **including** mistakes related to the amount and type of compounding ingredients. You have 6 minutes to complete this station.

Oral suspension of aluminum hydroxide antacid formula:

Aluminum hydroxide tablets	32.70 g
Sorbitol solution	28.20 mL
Syrup	9.30 mL
Glycerin	2.50 mL
Purified water, to make	qs to 100 mL

While you are watching, the pharmacy technician in training performed the following steps:

Step 1: She pulverizes the aluminum hydroxide tablets in a fine powder by trituration. She starts at the center of the mortar, with downward pressure on the pestle and a circular motion of very small diameter; rubs the product between the pestle and the mortar. Gradually increases the diameter of the circles until she reaches the side of the mortar and then decreases the diameter of the circles gradually until the center is again reached. She scrapes the powder frequently with a spatula from the sides of the mortar and from the bottom of the pestle. She continues the trituration until the desired particle size is attained.

Step 2: She adds 9.30 ml of syrup which acts as levigating agent to reduce further the particle size of aluminum hydroxide powder by continuing to grind in the mortar.

Steps 3: She adds 20 ml of purified water while stirring.

Step 4: She then adds 28.30 ml sorbitol solution and 2.50 ml glycerin while continuing to stir.

Steps 5: She transfers the mix in a dispensing bottled. Rinses the mortar and pestle with 10 ml purified waste and transfers the rinse solution to the dispensing bottle.

Step 6: She shakes the suspension to mix well.

Step 7: She adjusts the suspension to the desired volume of 100 ml with purified water

Answer Form - Compounding Skills Case #5

Procedures	Done accurately	Done incorrectly	Errors/omissions	Order the steps accurately
Step 1	O	O		
Step 2	O	Ⓞ	Syrup is not used as a levigating agent	
Step 3	O	O		
Step 4	O	O		
Step 5	O	O		
Step 6	O	O		
Step 7	O	O		

Answer Key – Compounding Skills Case #5

Procedures	Done accurately	Done incorrectly	Errors/omissions	Order the steps accurately
Step 1	●	O		Step 1
Step 2	O	●	Glycerin is used as levigating agent not syrup	Step 2
Step 3	●	O		Step 3
Step 4	●	O		Step 4
Step 5	●	O		Step 5
Step 6	●	O	Accurate by wrong order. Avoid shaking a suspension **during preparation** (refer to further learning below)	Step 7
Step 7	●	O	Wrong order.	Step 6

Further learning

Tips for preparing oral solutions and suspensions:

- Don't "qs" with a stirring rod in the container of oral liquid.
- Constantly stir when adding two liquids together.
- Stir smoothly and don't shake an oral liquid **during preparation** to avoid potential foaming
- Add high-viscosity liquids to less viscous liquids.
- Make sure that particle size of the active drug is reduced.

Tips for preparing emulsions:

- The drug must be added to the phase where it has the highest solubility
- Heat oily phase and its components
- Heat aqueous phase and its components few degrees above the temperature of oily phase
- Mix the two phases by adding the internal (small) phase to the external phase (large) while mixing
- Continue to mix vigorously until the mix cools and the emulsion sets

Compounding Suspensions

Beyond-Use Dating
The beyond-use date for a suspension should not be longer than 14 days, when refrigerated.
Auxiliary Labels
"Shake before using" is a common label used on suspension. Many will also require a "Refrigerate" label.

Compounding Solutions

Beyond-Use Date
The beyond-use date for solutions prepared from solid dosage forms shouldn't be more than 14 days from preparation, when refrigerated. The beyond-use date for elixirs can be up to six months.
Auxiliary Labels
For many compounded solutions, you will use a "Refrigerate" sticker.

Compounding Ointments

Beyond-Use Date
Generally, a 30-day beyond-use date should be assigned for ointments that do not contain water. For ointments that do contain water and no preservative, no more than a two-week supply should be dispensed. Ointments should generally be kept at room temperature.

Auxiliary Labels

Label ointments with "External use only."

Compounding Gels

Beyond-Use Date

Generally, water-containing gels should have a beyond-use date of no more than 14 days when stored at cold temperatures, such as in a refrigerator.

Auxiliary Labels

Label most topical gels with "External use only" and "Refrigerate."

Compounding Creams and Lotions

Beyond-Use Date

The beyond-use date for most creams and lotions if they contain water and are prepared from solid dosage forms will be 14 days when stored in the refrigerator.

Auxiliary Labels

Use the following auxiliary labels for most compounded creams and lotions:

- Refrigerate
- External use only
- Shake before using (lotions only)

Station #6: Preparation of an ointment

You are an experienced pharmacy technician responsible for training newly hired pharmacy technicians. Today, the pharmacy technician in training is demonstrating her compounding skills. She is preparing an aspirin ointment for pain according to the formula below. You are expected to evaluate her performance at each step. Use the **answer form** to record your findings by filling the circles and order the steps accurately if needed; if applicable, identify errors/omissions **including** mistakes related to the amount and type of compounding ingredients. You have 6 minutes to complete this station.

1% aspirin ointment formula:

Aspirin tablets 1 g
Oil-in-water emulsion base qs 100 g

While you are watching, the pharmacy technician in training performed the following steps:

Step 1: She triturates aspirin tablets using a mortar and pestle into a fine powder.
Step 2: She proceeds to incorporate the powder in 100 g hydrous lanolin of by levigation.
Step 3: She first places 100 g of hydrous lanolin on an ointment slab.
Step 4: She forms a well in the middle of the ointment base and adds aspirin powder.
Step 5: She mixes the two ingredients with a spatula with a slow steady motion starting from the center of well moving towards the edges.
Steps 6: Once the powder is entirely mixed, she continues to mix with the spatula until the ointment becomes homogenous.
Step 7: She transfers the ointment in a dispensing jar. The jar is labelled appropriately.

Answer Form - Compounding Skills Case #6

Procedures	Done accurately	Done incorrectly	Errors/omissions	Order the steps accurately
Step 1	O	O		
Step 2	O	O		
Step 3	O	Ⓞ	wrong drug	
Step 4	O	Ⓞ	need to do volumetric	
Step 5	O	Ⓞ	volumetric	
Step 6	O	O		
Step 7	O	O		

Answer Key – Compounding Skills Case #6

Procedures	Done accurately	Done incorrectly	Errors/omissions	Order the steps accurately
Step 1	●	O		Step 1
Step 2	O	●	Wrong choice of ointment base; hydrous lanolin is w/o. Examples of o/w ointment bases: Hydrophilic Ointment and Dermabase Wrong amount of ointment base, use 99g	Step 2
Step 3	●	O		Step 3
Step 4	O	●	Wrong procedure. Refer to the description of levigation below	Step 4
Step 5	O	●	Wrong procedure. Refer to the description of levigation below	Step 5
Step 6	●	O		Step 6
Step 7	●	O		Step 7

Further Learning

Preparation of ointments

The two methods used to prepare ointments are:

Spatulation or incorporation method: Triturate solid ingredients in a mortar until they are very fine. Then, in a mortar or on an ointment slab, make a paste of the powder with an equal amount of base. This is called **levigation.** Thoroughly mix the paste with another volume of base equal to that of the paste. Then continue this routine of mixing equal amounts of paste and base until the entire base has been added and you have a uniform preparation with a very small particle size. A mortar and pestle should be used for incorporating liquids into a base or for preparing larger quantities of an ointment.

Fusion method: The fusion method is particularly useful when solid waxes are included in the ointment to add viscosity. In this method, first melt the substance with the highest melting point by using a water bath but use as little heat as necessary. Then add the other ingredients on the basis of their decreasing melting points. When the entire mixture is liquefied, remove it from the water bath. Then stir the mixture until it congeals, to prevent possible separation and crystallization.

Station #7: Preparation of suppositories

You are an experienced pharmacy technician responsible for training newly hired pharmacy technicians. Today, the pharmacy technician in training is demonstrating his compounding skills. He is preparing sumatriptan suppositories for migraines according to the formula below. You are expected to evaluate his performance at each step. Use the **answer form** to record your findings by filling the circles and order the steps accurately if needed; if applicable, identify errors/omissions **including** mistakes related to the amount and type of compounding ingredients. You have 6 minutes to complete this station.

Sumatriptan suppository formula:

Sumatriptan 30 mg Cocoa butter qs 100% w/w Mft: sup #10

While you are watching, the pharmacy technician in training performed the following steps:

Step 1: He calculates the amount of sumatriptan, and cocoa butter needed to make 2 g (2000 mg) suppository. According to his calculation, he needs 23 mg of sumatriptan and 1,977 mg of cocoa butter assuming a gravity of sumatriptan in cocoa butter of 1.3

Step 2: He then calculates the amount of ingredients needed for the 10 suppositories. According to his calculation, he needs 230 mg of sumatriptan and 19,770 mg of cocoa butter.

Step 3: He slowly heats the 19,770 mg of cocoa butter to 40 ^{0}C while stirring.

Step 4: Once the cocoa butter is melted, he adds 230 mg of sumatriptan fine powder with mixing to disperse.

Step 5: He then pours slowly the mix in a 10 units suppository mold pre-lubricated with mineral oil. He ensures the mold is filled completely.

Step 6: He places the mold in the refrigerator to cool.

Step 7: Once the suppositories are set, he scraps excess from the mold. He then releases the suppositories.

Answer Form - Compounding Skills Case #7

Procedures	Done accurately	Done incorrectly	Errors/omissions	Order the steps accurately
Step 1	O	O		
Step 2	O	O		
Step 3	O	O		
Step 4	O	O		
Step 5	O	O		
Step 6	O	O		
Step 7	O	O		

Answer Key – Compounding Skills Case #7

Procedures	Done accurately	Done incorrectly	Errors/omissions	Order the steps accurately
Step 1	●	O		Step 1
Step 2	O	●	Add an **overage** of at least 2 suppositories to account for potential losses	Step 2
Step 3	●	O		Step 3
Step 4	●	O		Step 4
Step 5	O	●	Propylene glycol is preferred as lubricant for oleaginous bases like cocoa butter. Mineral oil is used for water soluble bases.	Step 5
Step 6	O	●	Allow the mold to set a room temperature to prevent cracks in the suppositories	Step 6
Step 7	●	O		Step 7

Station #8: Preparation of a solution

You are an experienced pharmacy technician responsible for training newly hired pharmacy technicians. Today, the pharmacy technician in training is demonstrating his compounding skills. She is preparing a solution of metronidazole according to the formula below. You are expected to evaluate his performance at each step. Use the **answer form** to record your findings by filling the circles and order the steps accurately if needed; if applicable identify errors/omissions **including** mistakes related to the amount and type of compounding ingredients. <u>You have 6 minutes to complete this station.</u>

Metronidazole solution formula

Metronidazole	1.0 g	cream colored powder	1 g/100 ml water; 0.5 g/100 ml ethanol; soluble in dilute acid	Antiprotozoal
HCl 10%	1.5 ml	clear, non-viscous liquid	miscible with water	Solubilizing agent
Propylene glycol	10.0 ml	clear, hygroscopic liquid	miscible with water	Solubilizing agent
Methylparaben	100 mg	white crystalline needles	1 g/400 ml water; 1 g/ 70 ml warm glycerol	Preservative
Propylparaben	50 mg	white crystal	soluble in 2000 parts water	Antifungal, preservative
Purified Water (solvent)			qs 100 ml	

While you are watching, the pharmacy technician in training performed the following steps:

Step 1. He makes methylparaben and propylparaben trituration.
Step 2. He adds methylparaben and propylparaben trituration to a scintillation vial and adds 10 ml propylene glycol. He shakes the vial until powders are dissolved.
Step 3. He adds the metronidazole to about 50 ml of purified water in a 100 ml beaker and begins stirring with a stir bar.
Step 4. He adds the hydrochloric acid solution to the beaker.
Step 5. He adds the methylparaben, propylparaben and propylene glycol mixture to the beaker. Rinse the scintillation vial with a few portions of purified water.
Step 6. He transfers the beaker contents to a pre-calibrated prescription bottle. He rinses the beaker with purified water and adds the rinse solution to the prescription bottle.
Step 7. He then adjusts the solution volume to 100 ml with purified water.

Answer Form - Compounding Skills Case #8

Procedures	Done accurately	Done incorrectly	Errors/omissions	Order the steps accurately
Step 1	O	O		
Step 2	O	O		
Step 3	O	O		
Step 4	O	O		
Step 5	O	O		
Step 6	O	O		
Step 7	O	O		

Answer Key – Compounding Skills Case #8

Procedures	Done accurately	Done incorrectly	Errors/omissions	Order the steps accurately
Step 1	●	O		Step 1
Step 2	●	O		Step 2
Step 3	●	O		Step 3
Step 4	●	O		Step 4
Step 5	●	O		Step 5
Step 6	●	O		Step 6
Step 7	●	O		Step 7

Station #9: Pharmaceutical Calculations

You are an experienced pharmacy technician responsible for training newly hired pharmacy technicians. Today, the pharmacy technician in training is demonstrating his pharmaceutical calculations skills. Calculating the correct amount of each ingredient is the first step in the process of compounding. You are expected to check the accuracy of calculated amount of compounding ingredients. Use the **answer form** to record your findings by filling the circles; if applicable, provide the accurate amount of ingredients. <u>You have 6 minutes to complete this station.</u>

Prescription order
Loratadine 10 mg
Pseudoephedrine 15 mg
Lactose 100 mg
Microcrystalline cellulose 24 mg
Magnesium stearate
Mft: 150 mg tab #200

The pharmacy technician's results are:
Calculation 1 - Total amount of powder in grams including10% excess (overage): **15 g**
Calculation 2 - Total amount of loratadine in grams including 10% overage: **2.0 g**
Calculation 3 - Total amount of pseudoephedrine in grams including 10% overage: **3.0 g**
Calculation 4 – The percentage strength of (w/w) of pseudoephedrine in each tablet: **10%**
Calculation 5 - The ratio strength for loratadine in each tablet: **1:1.5**

Answer Form - Compounding Skills Case #9

Compounding Ingredients	Correct	Incorrect	If incorrect, what is the correct value?
Calculation 1	O	O	
Calculation 2	O	O	
Calculation 3	O	O	
Calculation 4	O	O	
Calculation 5	O	O	

Answer Key – Compounding Skills Case #9

Compounding Ingredients	Correct	Incorrect	If incorrect, what is the correct value?
Calculation 1	O	●	150 mg x 200 tabs = 30g Add 30 g x 10% = 0.3g Total = 30.3 g
Calculation 2	O	●	10 mg x 200 tabs = 2000 mg = 2 g Add 2 g x 10% = 0.02g Total = 2.02g
Calculation 3	O	●	15 mg x 200 tabs = 3000 mg = 3 g Add 3 g x 10% = 0.03g Total = 3.03g
Calculation 4	●	O	15 mg/150 mg x 100% = 10%
Calculation 5	O	●	150 mg/10 mg =15 1 part loratadine per 15 parts total

Station #10: Pharmaceutical Calculations

You are an experienced pharmacy technician responsible for training newly hired pharmacy technicians. Today, the pharmacy technician in training is demonstrating her pharmaceutical calculations skills. Calculating the correct amount of each ingredient is the first step in the process of compounding. You are expected to check the accuracy of calculated amount of compounding ingredients. Use the **answer form** to record your findings by filling the circles; if applicable, provide the accurate amount of ingredients. <u>You have 6 minutes to complete this station.</u>

Prescription order
Phenobarbital 20 mg
Syrup NF 10% (v/v)
Glycerin 5% (v/v)
Alcohol 5% (v/v)
Methylparaben 0.1% (w/v)
Propylparaben 0.01% (w/v)
Water qs 5ml
Mft syrup dtd ii oz

The pharmacy technician's results are:
Calculation 1 – The amount of preparation to be dispensed: **50 ml** 60ml
Calculation 2 – The amount of a stock solution of phenobarbital 25mg/ml needed to fill the prescription: **12 ml**
Calculation 3 – The amount of syrup NF in grams needed to fill the prescription; the specific gravity of syrup NF is 1.3: **7.8 g**
Calculation 4 – The amount of phenobarbital in milligrams needed to fill the prescription:**240 mg**
Calculation 5 – Parts of methylparaben per parts of phenobarbital: **1 to 5**

Answer Form - Compounding Skills Case #10

Compounding Ingredients	Correct	Incorrect	If incorrect, what is the correct value?
Calculation 1	O	O	
Calculation 2	O	O	
Calculation 3	O	O	
Calculation 4	O	O	
Calculation 5	O	O	

Answer Key – Compounding Skills Case #10

Compounding Ingredients	Correct	Incorrect	If incorrect, what is the correct value?
Calculation 1	O	●	ii oz = 2 x 30 ml = 60 ml
Calculation 2	O	●	20 mg/5ml x 60 ml = 240 mg 240 mg x 1ml/25 mg = 9.6 ml of stock solution
Calculation 3	●	O	60 ml x (10 ml/100 ml) x 1.3 = 7.8 g
Calculation 4	●	O	20 mg /5ml x 60 ml = 240 mg **OR** 9.6 ml x 25 mg = 240 mg
Calculation 5	O	●	0.1g methylparaben/100 ml x 5 ml = 0.005 g = 5 mg 20 mg phenobarbital/5 mg methylparaben = 4 1 part methylparaben to 4 parts phenobarbital